Wisdom of aging

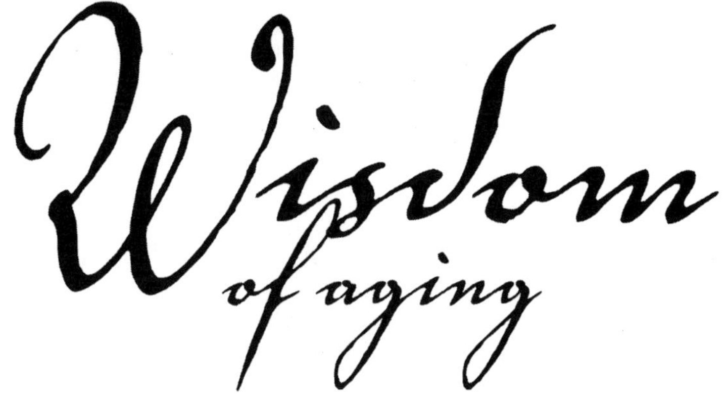

DORA O. CHIZEA, M.D.

Dora Chizea Productions
262 Lincoln Street, Ebensburg, Pennsylvania 15931

Copyright © 2002 by Dora O. Chizea, M.D.
All rights reserved
ISBN 0-9723818-0-5
Published by Dora Chizea Productions, 262 Lincoln Street, Ebensburg, Pennsylvania 15931

Disclaimer
This book is the author's personal view and theory. It is not intended to provide medical advice or to be used as a substitute for advice from the reader's personal physician.

"Age: Living in the Present Tense" (appendix), copyright © February 1991, The Christophers, Inc. Reprinted with permission of The Christophers, 12 East 48th Street, New York, NY 10017. This essay is an out-of-print Christopher News Note.

Dedication

This book is dedicated to all the Senior Citizens of Our Beautiful World.

Contents

Acknowledgments

I have no difficulty deciding where to begin or who to acknowledge first because even the most cursory reading of this book will reveal that I had a lot of help, what the world calls inspiration, from the Inspirer of Life and Source of all Knowledge and Wisdom.

I thank God for giving me the Holy Spirit, who literally dictated this book.

Next to God, I am always grateful to my Family. All the full and extended length, breadth and depth of it. The living and the transited members all. I hope I have reflected well the incredible love they seeded and nurtured in me. “Dalu nu.” (Thank you, all).

I acknowledge Sue Collins, the chronologically oldest but enthusiastically youngest nurse who worked with me while I was writing this book. She was most tolerant and accommodating of my countless requests to read my scripts and critique me as we went along. I wanted to get it right, and she was willing to help me do it. Thank you.

Others who must be mentioned for their patience with me in seeing that this book is produced, include my children, Chuchu, Ugo and Ebelem plus BolanLe Boglo, Kelechi Odu and Kanayo Oweazim. Though they were in their teenage years and early twenties, they were interested in “what the elders are reading!” and gave me useful tips. You make our beautiful tomorrow; and I say Thank you.

Dr. Ward Dean, M.D. a major researcher on vitamins and one of the originators of the Biological Aging concepts; did not know me when he read the brief on this book. His curiosity was stirred, and he wanted to know more. Once he knew more about my work, he gave me so much encouragement, it is hard to believe. He even directed me to sources that could help with the publication. He became a mentor and a friend just by caring. Thank you.

When I started this book, I did not know much about Dr. Mike Murdock, the television evangelist. Then one day I heard him talking about "Wisdom Keys" and realized that my book, *Wisdom of Aging,* was dealing with wisdom as a subject, just like he was. I began to take extra note of his presentations on our local television station. When I met him in person, I slipped the cover of my yet unfinished manuscript into his hand. That was giving him a preview and telling him, that I considered him a spiritual brother. Mike, thank you for being there.

Finally, I wish to thank my book agent, the publishers and all their staff who made it possible for this book to be in your hands today.

Thank you all.

Dora Obi Chizea, M.D.
Ebensburg, Pennsylvania

Introduction

This book is written with the objective of helping realign the Attitude to Aging held by so many people which makes it difficult for them to enjoy the Matured and Wisdom stage of their lives.

It is written to acknowledge the Fear, Anxiety and Negativism associated with aging, even when there is no active disease present and to replace these responses with Enjoyment, Confidence, Positivity and Wisdom that healthy longevity and aging offer.

It is a book written to help us find and define our position as we advance in age, in this changing world so that we can be present in mind and spirit to teach the next generation well.

So Rich

So Full

So Complete

The Cycle of Life

I hope you enjoy every bit of it before Transition Time.

Dora Obi Chizea, M.D

I

Conquer Your Fears

When you were young, most likely you could not wait to grow up, to leave home and begin making your own decisions. When you were young, you were strong, virile and daring. You knew everything. Well almost, so you thought. Your fears were only those of failure at school, work or play. But then you won more than you lost. And that was good enough. Your eyes were sharp, you could see clearly. Your hands were steady and you could thread any needle. Your ears were sharp, you could even hear the whispers of lovers from across the room. But you had your own lovers all around you, and it was not necessary to listen to others for long.

When you were young, your brain was sharp. You could learn and recall all new things, even trivia. It was exhilarating to soak in all that information and bounce around with new knowledge probably unknown to all before you. Your muscles were strong and your joints flexible. You could run and jump, twist and turn and dance all night. When you were young—that was before age thirty years—you were invincible.

But by age thirty your head was filled with stereotypical ideas about getting older. You want to "stop the clock," because you do not want to proceed any further in your physical journey. You have been told that the slope is down hill, and you are filled with fear. Fear of getting older and aging. Of losing your beauty. That you are not handsome enough any more. That the opposite sex does not find you attractive anymore. And when they do that your sexual prowess has lost its polish and vigor.

Your hair falls out when you comb it each morning, and it does not seem to grow back as fast. You fear you will become bald or that your baldness will get worse. You can live with little or no hair on your head. But then, you fear you will lose your brain and forget your friends' names. That you will lose your mind and walk out of the bathroom unzipped. That you will forget where you parked your car and walk around the parking lot in circles.

You fear you do not move fast enough, that everyone is passing you by. That if you walk faster you will fall down and break a hip. That nobody cares. That the youth have everything and they could care less.

Full of fear you are.

Then you find out that your age can expose you to the scourge of diseases. Arthritis that assaults your joints and leaves you with aches and pains that haunt your walking, sitting, and sleeping. High blood pressure that may bang up your heart with a heart attack and may even cause you a stroke and paralysis of body and limb.

Yes, you fear because it could be cancer that comes calling if dementia and Alzheimer's disease have not already made a Swiss cheese of your brain and made you a litter in an obscure corner of a nursing home. Yes, full of fear you are about aging.

So, what are you going to do about all these fears?

How Do You Get Your Fears?

Before we find out what you are going to do about these fears, we should explore how you got them. One thing we know for sure is that you were not born with fear. The human child has no fears. He is born a fearless explorer. Fear is a learned emotion. It is the negative feeling we get when we are anxious about the unknown. This unknown is usually in our future. Fear is a very powerful tool that can be manipulated to change attitude and behavior even when our rational mind and reality tell us differently.

The pharmaceutical manufacturers and the insurance gurus know about the power of fear so well that they use it as a tool to brainwash, bully and condition you into conforming with their plans to use you for their profit purposes.

For example, they give you statistics designed to make you anxious and fearful. They tell you that one in three men have ED, erectile dysfunction or impotence. That four million people in the U.S. have Alzheimer's disease and that this number may double by the year . That 40 million Americans have arthritis and pain. And that millions have cancer and on and on.

You are told that most of these things happen after age 50 or 65 years. Since every day you get closer to these numbers, you begin to look forward to those diseases and disabilities. And that is a fearful prospect.

We Become What We Expect

We become what we expect—well, not all the time, but more often than not. The bombardment with negative information about chances and risk of diseases like depression, heart disease, cancer and dementia paint a picture of gloom for people as they get older.

Over the years, these ideas get so ingrained into your psyche that you begin to expect one or more of these disorders to happen to you. This expectation creates your future and before you know it, the future is here.

A friend of mine always talks about when she gets old and is in a "rocking chair in the nursing home." She hopes her children will visit. Right there, you can see her vision of the future: sad, lonely and possibly abandoned. I told her to change the picture. She should see herself laughing and playing with her grandchildren, telling them stories about her own youth and possibly embellishing some of it.

"But that is not reality," she tells me.

"Reality is what you create by what you want," I reply. "As for me, I choose to be one happy, sharp and funky great grandmother, trading wits with my grand and great grandchildren, supporting charities, telling fabulous stories and sharing the wisdom of age. If all the men my age have not succumbed to ED—impotence, that is—I would definitely consider new loves."

"You got to be kidding," she says.

"I am not kidding," I reply. "And that's the way it is going to be."

II

Want to be a Millionaire? Think Like a Millionaire. Want to be Healthy? Think Healthy.

The principle of "If you want to become something, put your thoughts to it," does not apply to the youths only and it is not about money only. It applies to everyone including yourself. If you want to have healthy years ahead of you, you must not only think "healthy," you must also "act healthy."

For our purposes, forget everything that has happened to present. This is not judgment day. It is a new day of promise and hope. You begin the same way you teach the children. When you wake up in the morning, if you believe there is a God, say your prayers. Thank Him/Her for the past night and place the new day in His/Her hands. If you do not believe in God, you can do what you wish, but don't just go for the pot of coffee, bottle of gin or stick of cigarette or whatever to wake you up.

Sit up first in bed for a few seconds. Make sure you are not dizzy, then stand up. Make sure your feet are steady. If not, sit for a while and then try again, or hold onto something as you walk to the bathroom. Be sure to call your doctor and let him know if you had any problems waking up.

Next, brush your teeth with a strengthening and whitening tooth paste. If you do not like brushing, use dental powder or a soft chewing stick to clean your teeth. Do not feel offended, if you already do these things. Some people forget, so this is just a friendly reminder.

Before you brush or clean your teeth, always rinse out your mouth with water. This cleans out the film of bacteria and debris that may have accumulated in your mouth over night. Besides being good hygiene, this behavior may prevent you from some serious heart disease. Some experts believe that the plaque that thicken the arteries and cause arteriosclerosis or hardening of the arteries, are not from cholesterol, fats and calcium alone. They think that some bacterial infection are also involved in this process. Some of these bacteria come from the mouth. In fact, dentists usually encourage people who have some heart valve damage or heart murmur to take preventive antibiotics before dental work. If you brush your teeth without first rinsing out your mouth, thereby helping to reduce the bacterial load in your mouth, you increase your chances of showering your blood stream with bacteria, a state known as bacteremia, or bacteria in the blood. This could occur if your gum bleeds when you brush your teeth.

And that reminds me to say that if your gums bleed when you brush your teeth, take Vitamin C, or see the dentist to check you out for periodontal disease. If you take blood thinning medications like aspirin, warferin or gingko, you may have to cut back on your dosage or tell your doctor about it.

You should shower or bathe daily, not only to be clean but to wake your body and mind up. It could be in the morning or before going to bed. On cold days, take warm or hot showers or bath. And on warmer or hot days, take cold showers or bath.

Food

Eat according to your activity level. If you do heavy labor that require lots of calories, be sure to have a relatively high carbohydrate diet in the morning. If you are an executive, a student or some one who does a lot of calculations, eat a protein rich breakfast.

Whatever you do, eat breakfast to start your day. The amount of calories you take should not be more than you expend. Otherwise you will gain weight and burden your heart.

If you are already overweight, eat just fewer calories each day and eventually you will begin to notice some weight loss.

Everyone knows by now, that most nutritional experts recommend that you include lots of fiber, fresh vegetables and fruits in your daily meals. Avoid high fat diet if you can, especially animal fat.

Don't forget to take supplements of vitamins and minerals to keep your mind and body healthy.

Exercise and Music

You are almost always encouraged to exercise for about twenty minutes daily, but this can be misleading or impracticable as you get older. Usually, you are told to take a walk or climb stairs. I personally recommend that you play the music of your youth or any other music of your choice. The music you enjoyed and danced to as a teenager or young adult is very easy to get into as you age. It could be the Twist, Rock 'n' Roll, The Jerk, Hip Hop, whatever.

If you have your own place, play your music there, if not, use an ear phone. Spend at least one hour each day listening to, dancing to, or tapping to it. It raises your spirit, makes you feel good and often stimulates you into the dance of your youth and the healthy vibrations associated with the period. Don't think anyone is going to laugh at you. If they do, simply invite them to join you in the music and dance. It's aerobics. Sure you can tread mill and do a whole variety of exercise, but your personal music added to it makes it so much more fun.

Rest and Quiet Time

Physical, mental and emotional rest is important for your good health. You have to program it into your daily life. I heard this from a television program one evening. I do not remember the name of the speaker but she was from the Caribbean Islands. She was a lady in her 80s lecturing on rest. She said that when she was a little girl, her mother used to say: "Five hours sleep is all you need, girl. Eight hours is too much. Ten hours is wickedness!"

I thought that was great. The message is that five to eight hours sleep a day will keep you healthy. If you sleep too long, you begin to lose the benefit of rest and reap the harvest of laziness and degeneration of your joints and muscles. Long hours of sleep may also indicate that you are depressed or have low thyroid hormone. See your doctor if this is the case.

I also recommend a fifteen to sixty minute nap or quiet time during the day. It may be at your lunch time or after work. This should be your "quiet/private time" when you let your mind "do nothing." Just let the mind wander as it pleases. If you know the art of meditation or yoga this can be a time to practice them. These "quiet/private times" are your refreshment and refueling time for your mind and spirit and they help to restore your total health. Use your quiet time to visualize yourself in good health, happy, fulfilled in the future and fantasize on the legacy you will leave behind for your family and friends or even the world at large.

Now, let us tackle the fear of dementia and Alzheimer's before we talk about how to age with a purpose.

III

Alzheimer's: This, Too, Shall Pass

Though Alzheimer's Dementia is said to affect only 4 million of the 274 million in the U.S., its negative image as the destroyer of human memory looms menacingly over the baby boomers like a dark shadow.

A short while ago, one of our friends in her early 50s was diagnosed with Alzheimer's. This came as distressing news to myself and my friends. Four of us, two men and two women, Tom, Joe, Anna and myself, between 40 and 55 years, decided to brainstorm on what we were going to do for our friend and ourselves. Three of us were very vocal, but Joe said nothing. He just sat with a sad distant look in his eyes. He nodded periodically but said nothing throughout the two hours we spent together that afternoon. Joe was usually the most talkative of us all, but he was so deeply affected, he was speechless.

Tom, on the other hand, was very anxious for us to do something for our friend, but he felt helpless. With deep emotions, eyes clouded with tears and a quivering voice, Tom told us that he had just buried his father, a victim of Alzheimer's.

You Don't Wish Alzheimer's Even on Your Worst Enemy

"You don't wish Alzheimer's even on your enemy," he said. "It is a most devastating disease. My father died in my arms, but he wasn't even present at his own death. He was long gone before he passed on." He then relayed to us the deep sad story of his father's and family's experience. "Alzheimer's is not a one person's disease. It is a family's tragedy," he told us. To watch a previously independent loved one go from forgetting his car keys to not remembering his own home address, not recognizing his wife and children is sad. To see him screaming and crying for no obvious reason, wandering and getting lost is heart breaking. But for him to end up unable to brush his teeth, comb his hair, or even use the toilet by himself is the bottom of humiliation.

Tom told us that his father lost his language and forgot how to talk. "At his death, he could barely say 'Dada' like a baby." By this time, tears were streaming down his eyes uncontrollably. He did not say so, but it was obvious that Tom was afraid for himself too. If Alzheimer's is supposed to be partially genetic, statistics has it that Tom has a 50 percent chance of getting it eventually as a first degree relative of his father.

Was that his future?

We all sat for a while in silence, each in his/her own thought. "So what are we going to do to prevent this devastation?" Anna quietly nudged us on with our meeting. "Tania is only 52 years old. I don't understand what's happening. I thought you are not supposed to get this disease until you are much older, like in your eighties, well maybe age 65 at least. Is there anything we can do to slow it down?" Anna looked askance at me, the one with the medical background.

What is Alzheimer's Disease?

"Alzheimer's disease is a progressive mental condition produced by excessive brain cell destruction and death. The disease takes 8 to 10 years to progress, and it can take as much as 20 years to ultimately terminate in death. Over these years, the brain shrinks in size. This cell loss leads to memory loss, difficulty learning, difficulty retaining information, and difficulty accessing old information like the name of the person's high school." I started my dissertation.

As we could see from Tom's story, Alzheimer's disease affects one's mood, personality and behavior. Delusions, hallucinations, aggression and wandering also occur and by death time, the person is usually regressed to the stage of a helpless baby.

What Is Wrong with the Brain?

Before we can do something about it, we must take a few moments to understand what has gone wrong to make the brain cells die. You see, just as our skin sloughs and regrows and just as our hair cuts, falls and re-grows, the brain like any other organ/ tissue in the body is constantly changing, recycling and renewing itself. If our skin sloughs and new skin grows to replace it, our skin will always be fresh and healthy. But if our skin sloughs as we age and it is not renewed and replaced, then it will thin out and possibly have holes or wrinkles on it.

The same is true of our brain. The chemicals in the cells of the brain called neurotransmitters which handle messages within the brain and which send messages to and from the brain are constantly being recycled and used up. But they are also constantly being re-manufactured and replaced to maintain the health of the brain.

If for any reason these chemicals are used up or destroyed and are not replaced, then with time, the amount of chemicals needed to do the brain work of thinking, remembering, planning, and behaving will not be enough and the person will begin to have a decrease or loss of these brain functions. This person will be said to be demented. The process is known as dementia, meaning decreased mental energy.

Meanwhile, to continue the skin analogy, we know that as we get older, though, we continue to replenish our sloughed skin, the replacement is never quite perfect, so the skin texture and flexibility we have as adults is not the same as the skin we had as babies.

By the same token, as we get older, our brains are not as flexible and pliable as a child's, and we are not able to learn and retrieve information as well as young people do. This happens because time and age in general decrease the brain cells' chemical productions. As we get older, we produce fewer of the neurotransmitters that we need for thinking, remembering, learning and behaving.

Age-associated loss of brain function is sometimes called Senile Dementia or Age Associated Memory Loss. Some people consider this as part of normal aging like gray hair. It need not be so.

There are many causes of dementia, including environmental pollution, head injury, stress, cardiovascular (heart and blood vessel) diseases, disarrayed immune system, Down's Syndrome, and the female sex after menopause. But family and genetic predisposition, is by far (50 percent of all dementia) the commonest.

So, in answer to Anna's, "What are we going to do?" I said, "Mental Hygiene and the Brain Preservation Program."

Here is what you can do to keep your brain generally healthy and keep the gene of Alzheimer's from expressing itself if you happen to be a carrier of such a gene.

IV

Mental Hygiene and Brain Preservation Program

Remember syphilis?

Remember polio?

Remember smallpox?

Remember AIDS?

They were all scourges that came and passed or at least were subjugated. Alzheimer's Dementia (AD), too, will pass. We are in the midst of very active research that will soon enough make AD a history book disorder. So, relax and practice your Mental Hygiene and Brain Preservation Program.

The first objective of this program is to limit Age Associated Dementia and prevent AD from expressing itself. The second objective is to restore brain health.

There are seven steps in this program.

1. Diet and Nutritional Management
2. Stress Management
3. Physical and Mental Exercise
4. Life-style Changes
5. Pharmaceutical Management
6. Herbal Management
7. Family Love

Diet and Nutrition

Like most people, you may have struggled with your diet and nutrition at some point in your life. Most of that struggle is usually about gaining or losing weight, having the ideal body weight, size and shape so that you can put on clothes that flatter you.

It is not very often that people consciously say to themselves, "I am going to eat a brain healthy food today." But that is what you have to do if you want your brain to have an abundance of the neurotransmitters and the energy you need to remain alert, continue to learn new things, service your memory store, and maintain your dignity.

You have to be sensible about what you put in your mouth. Don't eat just because you are hungry. Anticipate your hunger and plan your meals in such a way that you will always have brain healthy foods around you.

First of all eat real foods rather than junk foods. Buy them, whenever you can, from the grocery produce section of your supermarket, rather than from the frozen or pre-cooked and instant food section.

The fuel or energy supply for the brain is sugar. You must not starve your brain of sugar by starvation diets that put you in hypoglycemic (low blood sugar) states, because it can decrease the brain function and can lead to damage and even death of brain cells that will bring you closer to dementia.

While you should avoid hypoglycemia, do not take your sugars in "free" form like table sugar, syrups and soda pops. These free sugars destabilize your blood sugar balance by stimulating excessive insulin release which has its own complications. It is best to take in your sugars in the form of complex sugars, called carbohydrates. Rice, pasta and potatoes are examples of carbohydrates. If you supply your body with small amounts of carbohydrates every four to six hours during the day, the brain will have enough fuel energy to do its job.

Eat a Balanced Diet

You need to eat a balanced diet because the brain and the whole body need all the ingredients to be available in order to produce the balanced and good health you want as you progress in age. Include whole grains in the form of cereal, bread, and baked foods in your daily meal. Vegetables and fruits should also be eaten daily. Low-fat meat or poultry, low-fat dairy, fish, and plant proteins like soy and beans should be part of your diet. It is from these proteins that the amino acids are made. Amino acids are the building blocks for the production of neurotransmitters, the brain messengers without which the brain becomes dysfunctional.

You should also take supplements of vitamins and minerals daily. They are important as co-factors (enablers), which accelerate or control the utilization of the other nutrients in the body. Magnesium deficiency (low blood magnesium level), for example, is common in Alzheimer's Dementia. Daily supplementation with magnesium is important for brain health. In fact, there are several other vitamins and minerals important for your brain health but rather than make a list of them, I suggest that you find a good source of multivitamins with minerals, and take one daily.

Make sure that your daily supplement includes all the eight amino acids which your body needs, but which cannot be manufactured by the body, so they have to be taken into your body as food. You need not know their names, but they are tryptophan, lysine, isoleucine, leucine, methionine, phenylalanine, valine, and threonine. You really only need to check that the label of your high potency multivitamin and minerals also say plus the essential amino acids. If not, find additional sources for these important nutrients like lean meat, turkey, fish and soy.

Vitamin B complex is important for the integrity of your brain and nervous system so be sure to take one tablet of Mega B-Complex or at least B-50 each day. This will automatically include folic acid, which belongs to the B-Complex family.

Do not forget the antioxidants Vitamin E 400 I.U. daily, Vitamin C 500 -1000 mg once or twice daily and Vitamin A (Beta Carotene) 5,000 -15,000 I.U. daily.

A powerful antioxidant made from hydrogen with an extra ion on it called microhydrin will boost your antioxidant status in ways that feels like magic. One or two capsules a day will make you feel so much better mentally and physically, too. Add this to your regimen if you can, you will be glad you did.

Add to these, chromium picolinate 200mcg/day to help keep your blood sugar in balance and keep the brain well fueled. Selenium 100 - 200 mcg/day will help keep your immune system working well, and that means fighting against age-related diseases like cancer, heart disease and stroke which can cause dementia.

N-acetyl cysteine 150 - 500 mg, lecithin (soy) 1200mg, Acetyl l-carnitine 500mg, and fish oil concentrate with omega-3 fatty acids 1000mg are additional supplements for a healthy brain and body.

Co-enzyme Q-10 is usually regarded as a supplement for your heart and blood vessels. True. But remember that good blood circulation is also important for the brain. So a brain-healthy supplementation should include Co-enzyme Q-10 100 mg/ day.

This is all I am going to say about nutrition for healthy brain at this point. There are many books on good nutrition and several web sites where you can learn about the countless options you have.

The message for now is that you should plan your eating with your brain's health in mind and eat for life and good health and not for death and degenerative diseases. Enjoy what you eat. If you do not enjoy it, don't eat it. You are old enough to make that decision.

V

Stress Management for Brain Health

Most people know that stress is not good for them. What many people are not quite sure of is how very bad chronic stress can be for the brain.

I have a little book, *Link-Up: A New Paradigm for Stress and Stress Management in the New Millennium*, which I recommend you read, if you have not already read it. It deals with what chronic stress does to the whole body. For now we are going to see how chronic stress can cause dementia and possibly exacerbate Alzheimer's Disease.

Norepinephrine (NEpi), one of the four major neurotransmitters (NT) involved in Alzheimer's and other dementias, is well known as a major stress hormone involved in the "Fight and Flight Response." By the way, the other three NTs are dopamine, acetylcholine and seratonin. But we are not going to discuss those three now.

Norepinephrine (NEpi) is a major NT involved in long-term memory. Have you ever wondered how come you remember some events in your past, especially in your childhood, very vividly, while you can hardly remember some of the other events that occurred at about the same period, even with prompting?

I recall that as children, we used to raid the pear tree in the compound of an elderly gentleman in our town. As kids, we thought he was a miser because his tree was always laden with fruits and he never seemed to eat them and never gave them away to us kids. Those pears were delicious, we thought.

Adventure

On one occasion, half a dozen of us kids decided to raid the pear tree and pick as many fruits as we could. We knew that if the old man caught us, we could be in trouble. Our raiding team decided that since I was an agile tree climber, I should climb the tree and shake the branches vigorously so that the ripe pears would fall, and the rest of the team on the ground would pick up as many as they could and run away before the old man came out screaming, "Stupid kids! Stupid kids!"

So off we went at dusk, because we needed some darkness to hide so that if the old man came out and found us, he would not be able to recognize us and report us to our parents.

Excitement

Well, when we got there, I jumped on the tree like a squirrel and before you could say "Twinkle, Twinkle Little Star," I was shaking every branch of tree in my path and the pears were tumbling down while my friends gathered them as fast as they could. Then suddenly: Silence!

Before the silence could register in my mind, all my friends had disappeared. Then I heard the most chilling voice I had ever heard, "I know you are up there, and I am going to be sitting right here when you come down!"

I froze onto the branch of the tree next to me. I was in paralysis. I could not afford to breathe because the old man was holding his shot gun.

I knew he could not stand under the tree for very long because he had a bad leg. I kept holding my breath in what seemed like an eternity. Then as I watched the old man try to find a spot to sit down, I jumped off the tree in a flash like lightning and disappeared into the engulfing darkness. Before the old man's reflexes could react, I was gone. Safely out of danger, my heart jumped and pounded like it was going to leave my body.

Was that stress or what!

Need I say that was the last raid of my life!

Acute Stress Release Norepinephrine

Why do I remember this incident so vividly? I was eight years old at the time. I do not remember other things that happened to me that year. Why? Because the large outpouring of the neurotransmitter and acute stress mediator norepinephrine etched that traumatic and exciting event in my long-term memory store.

It is for this same reason that you remember your own childhood trauma, special events, abuses (sexual or otherwise) and great victories and disappointments.

You see, it is the job of norepinephrine to help us record exciting or traumatic and emotional events that occurred a long time ago. Norepinephrine is an energizing chemical, a happiness chemical that elevates your mood and keeps you optimistic. It is the neurotransmitter of zest. When norepinephrine is low you cannot lay down and store your long term memory properly; your mood is depressed and you feel sad. Low norepinephrine makes it difficult for you to concentrate on any task and impossible to cope with stress.

So now, you see why norepinephrine is very important for your brain health. If you do not have enough norepinephrine either because you are not making enough of it or because the brain cells that should be using it have been destroyed by trauma or disease, you forget to remember your past and may even forget the name of your high school.

Coping with Acute Stress

Everyone knows that when you are acutely stressed with fear or anxiety you may become irritable, confused or even panic-stricken and irrational. You need norepinephrine, among other things, to cope with the "fight-flight-freeze-faint" response that the acute stress brings. Norepinephrine is made from amino acids, especially tyrosin and phenylalanine. Amino acids come from proteins in the food you eat.

If you include high-protein sources like poultry, dairy and soy products in your nutritional therapy as discussed above you should have a head start for dealing with acute stress.

The proteins do not work alone. They need the help of folic acid, magnesium, Vitamin C and B-12. This is one of the reasons for recommending that you include a good multivitamin source, B-Complexes, minerals and essential amino acids in your daily healthy brain nutrition.

Chronic Stress and Brain Health

While acute stress is handled by Norepinephrine and other chemicals, chronic stress is a different problem altogether. With chronic stress you lie awake night after night worrying about the bills, school fees, mortgage, car payment, food, clothing, club dues and so on. You worry about your image and the impression you are making on your boss, co-workers, colleagues, and society at large and you are consumed by it. When you live in fear and anxiety about arguing or fighting with your spouse or partner, you are under chronic stress.

You are no longer in the stage of "fight-flight-freeze-faint" response. You are in the long-term "What am I going to do?" state. Cortisol is the chemical that handles this state of your being. The first intentions of the body, in this case the adrenal glands, in releasing cortisol to come to the acutely stressed body that is becoming overwhelmed by worry, anxiety or fear, is good.

In the beginning cortisol helps the brain in two ways. First, it helps to ensure that the stressed brain does not run out of fuel (glucose). It does this by breaking down protein and converting it into sugar in a chemical process called gluconeogenesis. It also decreases the utilization of sugar by all the other organs of the body so that the brain can have as much fuel as it needs to cope with the challenge being faced.

These are good deeds indeed. But when cortisol persists in its protein breakdown task, it begins to destroy vital systems of the body that are protein dependent. For example, the immune system is weakened and even the brain cells (neurons) in the hippocampus are damaged. And these hippocampal neurons (brain cells) are the ones whose death result in Alzheimer's disease!

So there!—for cortisol's help in chronic stress! Persisting elevated cortisol in chronic stress is actually toxic to the brain cells. Excess cortisol decreases attention span. It makes it difficult for one to focus. It makes long term learning difficult and reduces the speed with which one processes memory and information. For example, while attempting to recall an event in the past, you find your mind getting stuck.

You can't quite recall the sequence of an event. You have doubts. "Was it Peter or John who came to visit us that day?" you ask your partner. And then you don't remember if he came alone or with someone else.

A chronically stressed, cortisol intoxicated brain, suffers from progressively decreasing memory, decreased learning ability and general loss of cognition. You begin to lose your mind.

No, you do not want to lose your mind. You do not want to be intoxicated with cortisol. No, you do not want to be under the grips of chronic stress.

Reducing Cortisol Intoxication

First of all, I will again encourage you to read my book, *Link-Up,* as noted earlier on. It discusses some very important stress coping skills that you might find useful if you do not already have those skills.

Also, there are several other books including Dr. Herbert Benson's *Relaxation Response* which may be of help to you.

However, one of the best and fastest ways to decrease the outpouring of cortisol is by caring for and nurturing someone, petting an animal or being petted yourself. You may not recall your own childhood, but in your life you must have come across a little baby lying alone on a crib crying. The crying and fusing invariably continues, once started, until the parent or a caregiver picks the baby up and holds him close to their body. This is an act of nurturing that calms the baby, removes his anxiety, whatever it might have been and tells him everything is all right.

Do you recall, even as adult, how it feels having someone hug you or place his/her hand on your shoulder to reassure you of their presence and care? That is nurturing and it brings the cortisol level of chronic stress down. The simple human act of grooming your child, spouse, friend or parent bring the toxic cortisol levels down. These acts are good for your brain's health and for preventing dementia and Alzheimer's. They keep the chronic stress chemical levels down and prevent cortisol from frying your brain.

VI

Nurturing Need for Brain Health

Loneliness is stressful. You can sleep on the same bed with your spouse and still be lonely. You can live with ten people in your house and still be lonely. You can work with a dozen people in your place of work and still be lonely. You can go to church, the temple or mosque with hundreds of people and still be lonely. You can live in a small town or big city and still be lonely.

Loneliness is a state in which there is a lack of ability to be open and vulnerable to share caring and nurturing which can only be transcribed by human contact (hugging, holding, touching, massaging or grooming).

Unfortunately, loneliness is the current state of the world because the modern person has been conditioned into feeling that human nurturing and human physical contact with an adult is a sign of weakness or a perverse sexual act. People are averse to touching and feeling one another because they do not want to be labeled gay, queer or "funny."

Yet we are all crying out for caring and nurturing deep inside our core. We long for human contact because imprinted somewhere in our DNAs is the knowledge that if we do not have human nurturing contact, the cortisol level in us will rise and fry our brains to dementia and Alzheimer's.

But the socio-techno-cultural milieu that we now live in say we should not nurture adults or allow ourselves to be nurtured.

In the loneliness that ensues, we go to chat rooms on the internet to seek faceless companionship. But that is only an illusion of human contact. Our need for physical nurturing remains unfulfilled and so we turn to drugs for further delusion.

We carry labels of social phobia, generalized anxiety disorder, bipolar disorder and depression among other names to cover our misplaced aversion for us, human beings. We push more drugs down our throat, up our nose and other orifices. We paste them as skin patches or rub them all over our skin. In one futile way or the other we try to fill our need for nurturing.

How very sad for us all in society, and especially the elders, who for one excuse or other have the least nurturing. They get tossed into nursing homes when their cortisol ravaged brains have been thoroughly punctured with holes we call Alzheimer's. But it need not be so.

Choose to Nurture Others and be Nurtured Yourself

We are told by experts that the number of people with dementia and Alzheimer's is rising though they are not quite sure why. They speculate that since the Baby Boomer Generation are getting into their fifties and racing into retirement and old age, if nothing is done to prevent and control dementia and Alzheimer's as many as eight million adults in the USA alone will be in the grips of Alzheimer's by the year 2025.

But the U.S. is not the only country with baby boomers. Almost every country that went to war during the second World War has the baby boom phenomenon. The U.S. is also not the only country with chronic stress induced hyper-cortisolism.

This section of my message is for any human being who is already aging or who will age at some point in the future, regardless of their geographic location on planet Earth.

You Have a Choice

You can choose to nurture people around you and be nurtured yourself also, or you can say, "Big boys and girls don't cry," act tough and pay for it later with a moth eaten brain.

You have a choice to say "No" to the idea that if you hug your child or grandchild or your friend's or neighbor's child or grandchild you are sexually stimulating them and the law enforcement agents will be knocking at your door soon with accusation of child molestation.

You have the choice to say "No" to the idea that being lonely, as discussed above, is a sign of your independence. Unfortunately, loneliness is against nature's protocol and will exert a toll on your brain.

You have the choice to say "No" to the idea that sex is the same thing as nurturing. Sex is a chemical and physical phenomenon; nurturing is a spiritual phenomenon; it is only on rare occasions that the two intersect. There is a whole section on "Love, Sex and Aging" in this book and more clarification will be given there.

You have the choice to say "No" to the idea that caring and nurturing is a sign of weakness and should be left to women, children, weak men and paid servants. Caring and nurturing are actually edifying and empowering for those who give.

Old Enough for a Revolution

You are old enough to lead a revolution at least in your own life. Here is a small revolution you can try.

You can choose to say "Yes" to the age-long practice of humans, as parents and caring adults by picking up your child, grandchild or your friend's or neighbor's child or grandchild, putting him or her on your lap, and telling a story, a joke or just have a chat with him or her. Ask the child what he or she is learning in school and discuss it, if you have some idea, or ask the child to educate you more about his more current information.

If you are too frail to pick them up, or if they are too big to be picked up by you, have them sit near you. Touch them, talk to them. It is for this reason that you are still alive, to nurture and teach the next generation.

You can also choose to say "Yes" to baby sitting or mentoring programs for the young in your community, YWCAs, schools, churches, playgrounds and wherever the opportunity or need arises.

You can say "Nonsense" to aversion to other adult human beings. Hug them, kiss them, hold their hands, roughhouse with them, cry with them, dance with them, embrace them, give them a back rub and receive the same from them.

You can choose to "Stop" thinking and feeling badly about other people whom you may not agree with but who are trying in their own way to lower their own cortisol levels by ostensibly caring for and nurturing other adults regardless of their gender, race, color or creed. Every one's DNA demands nurturing; otherwise the brain is made to pay heavily for its lack in stressful degeneration.

In the conclusion to this book we discuss Universal Love, which gives us self worth as expressed in nurturing. There can be no nurturing without human contact.

VII

Physical and Mental Exercise for Brain Preservation

Just about everyone knows the adage, "If you don't use it, you lose it." The brain is one organ that this adage fits to the T.

As they get older, some people abandon themselves. They do nothing to make their aging an asset. They make little or no effort at enhancing their physical and mental well being. This self abandonment leads to physical and mental weakness, slower physical and mental agility and general clumsiness in many physical and mental activities. Of course, this can lead to fall and various handicaps, but that is another issue for another time. For now, we are interested in the effects of physical exercise on mental health.

Physical Exercise and Brain Health

You are probably familiar with the benefits attributed to physical exercise. You know for example, that moderate aerobic exercise program can help reduce weight in the overweight, firm the body, enhance the muscle outlines and so improve the physical profile, make clothes fit better, lower elevated blood pressures and so on.

What you may not be so familiar with is that physical exercise can also improve brain health and performance. Moderate physical exercise helps to increase the oxygenation of your brain cell, increase your mental alertness, make your thinking process faster and clearer, improve your sleep and sense of well being.

It also helps to normalize and balance the all important brain chemicals (neurotransmitters), making you less prone to brain deteriorating conditions, decreases anxiety, alleviates depression, elevates mood and lowers dangerous cortisol level.

Now you know why you must get up and start moving, no matter how minimally and modestly you begin.

Mental Exercise

While physical exercise is good for your brain, mental exercise is even better and more specific for your functional brain health. It increases the oxygen and sugar (glucose) that goes to and is utilized by the brain. It also clears the brain of waste products of metabolism.

Mental exercise increases your ability to learn new things, retrieve past information or data more easily and become more imaginative and creative. It makes you more alert, focused and optimistic in outlook. The stimulation of mental exercise makes your brain grow in size and content even when you are already advanced in chronological age. It encourages your brain cells (neurons) to sprout more branches (dendrites) to reach out to other neurons and increase the speed and universality of the message being transmitted and shared. Mental exercise also helps the brain recover from injuries like concussions, mini strokes and even major strokes sometimes.

At the end of this book is a list of references of publications where you may find the scientific proofs for these claims about the positive effects of mental exercise, if you want to learn more about this subject. For now and for our purposes, I am going to discuss some of the mental exercises that are helpful for any brain, not only for the aging brain.

Recall that at the beginning of this section we quoted the adage, "If you don't use it, you lose it." Well, if you do not use your brain, just as if you do not use your muscles, it shrinks. Yes, the brain shrinks if it is not made to work.

The work of the brain is to record, store, interpret, and transcribe information; recognize and retrieve stored information, organize old and new information, release information, make decisions and instruct the rest of the body on what to do and how to act or behave. You have to challenge the brain daily for it to retain its plasticity and versatility.

There are many things you can do daily or periodically to stimulate or challenge your brain, but the most important thing is that you must like and enjoy it. If you are a mathematician who is poor in language, don't frustrate yourself with attempting to learn a new language as a way of challenging or exercising your brain. Play mathematical games instead. And if you are a linguist, begin to learn another language that will keep your brain busy and exercised.

Daily reading of newspapers and magazines, watching the evening news to learn about what is happening around you and in the world at large will help keep your brain active. Thought-provoking discussions with family, friends and colleagues participation in quiz games and problem solving on TV or in your family, and even cross word puzzles will keep the oxygen and sugar flowing into your brain cells.

Drawing, writing, teaching your child or grandchild or mentoring someone else's child will keep your brain exercised for sure. Just think of all the "Why This and Why That?" you have to answer when the kids are around. You can also play games like chess and scrabble, creative games like painting, sculpturing and construction of models with your peers or with younger persons.

There is a particular mental exercise I enjoy and recommend and that is to write down one wise saying from your life's experience every day, preferably at breakfast time and to re-read and contemplate that saying when you are going to bed. If you can add meditation and possibly some form of yoga at some point in your day or week, you can be sure that your brain will be as sharp as a razor blade. The youth will seek you out because your words will become an illustration of another adage: "Words of our Elders are Words of Wisdom."

Yes, you must preserve your brain because the next generation needs wisdom, and that cannot be downloaded from the computer. Wisdom comes from the dynamics of the human intellectual interplay on the fertile soil of a nurtured mind. We maintain these dynamics through physical and mental exercises for brain health.

VIII

Life-Style Changes for Brain Health

Life-style changes for our brain health are any new options we introduce into our behavior and daily practices to replace the pre-existing behavior and practices that are detrimental to the optimal functioning of our brain. They are behavioral changes introduced to impact your brain's health positively enough to reverse, retard and prevent brain degeneration. In many instances, they may enhance your mental acuity and productivity.

In addition to all the nutrients we discussed earlier, a healthy brain needs constant supply of oxygen and glucose to function properly. It requires that its waste disposal system, the blood circulation, remains patent and efficient. It also needs rest, relaxation and restoration of its neurons. Any behavior or practice which interferes with these processes will be detrimental to the healthy functions of the brain. And any behavior or practice that augments any or all of these processes will enhance the healthy functions of the brain.

Life-Style 1

Let us examine some life-styles (behaviors and practices) that may affect the oxygen supply to the brain.

Smoking is an example of a practice that robs the brain of adequate oxygen supply. It is not surprising, therefore, that smoking is sometimes implicated in some dementias and strokes.

Life-Style Change 1

A good life-style change, if you smoke, would be to stop smoking. The extra oxygen you save might be helpful in your brain longevity efforts.

Life-Style 2

Another example is the continuous consumption of fatty foods and highly refined sugar products. They can lead to arteriosclerosis, that is, the clogging up of the blood circulation to the heart and other vital organs including the brain. This clogging up of the blood supply to the brain, can lead to decreased oxygen supply to the brain and accelerate the damage to and loss of brain cells and function. In some cases, strokes and paralysis can even result.

Life-Style Change 2

A life-style change, in this case, could be to change your eating habits if you have been eating excessive fatty and highly refined sugar products. You could begin to eat meals that have less fat and less sugar. Including fresh fruits, vegetables, lean meats, fish, and complex carbohydrate as previously discussed would probably be more healthy for your brain.

Life-Style 3

The excessive use of alcohol and drugs, especially mind altering drugs, interfere with the cells of the brain (neurons) damaging them and sometimes killing them. In addition to being toxic to the brain (neurotoxic), alcohol and drugs, can impede the waste disposal function of the kidneys with detrimental consequences to the whole body. When the brain is immersed in toxic waste, it makes the mind foggy, perceptions distorted, and imagination deluded instead of the mind being clear, sharp and astute.

Life-Style Change 3

A suggested life-style change, if you use excessive alcohol or abuse drugs, would be to stop this behavior. But it may not be very easy to stop, so you may need to see your doctor or seek counseling for assistance.

Life-Style 4

Seclusion, loneliness, and avoiding human interaction are behaviors or life-styles that prevent your brain from being stimulated and challenged. As discussed above, when your brain is not challenged or stimulated, it shrinks and loses function.

Life-Style Change 4

A life-style change that will help in this example would be to seek interactive activities such as conversations, discussions, and games that involve other people.

Rest, Relaxation and Restoration Time for the Brain

The brain needs rest, relaxation and restoration to recharge itself and be in the shape for optimal productivity.

When I was a little girl I was involved in several extra curricular activities. I was in the girl guides society, debating society, science society and writing club. I was also a potential Olympic Athlete who had to do my athletic practice daily.

But over and above all, I wanted good grades so I would be able to go to medical school someday.

As you can imagine there were never enough hours in a day for me to complete everything I wanted to do each day. My brain was young and pliable then, but I would have been stressed out if my father had not taught me how to "power nap." He taught me how to take ten minutes in the middle of the day and just close my eyes, let go every thought or imagination in my head and just be. When I opened my eyes ten minutes later, I felt brand new.

In support of my boarding school authorities, my father also encouraged me to take a siesta break for at least forty-five minutes after school hours before beginning my home work or my extra curricular activities. He insisted that I had a minimum of five hours' sleep every night, though sometimes I got away with four hours' sleep if I had to study for an exam or had special tasks to accomplish. I have pretty much practiced what I was taught in childhood and have passed on the same kind of wisdom to my own children.

The message is that we need rest, relaxation and restoration for brain health. If you have a life-style that keeps you on the run, slow down. Find time to rest, relax and restore your mental equilibrium so that you do not lose your mind to cortisol and stress.

There is so much that can be said about life-style changes for healthy brain but this is all we can take for now. The references at the end of this book will give you more resources to review, if you are inclined to read more about it.

Now, we are ready to look at the pharmaceutical aids available for mental hygiene and brain preservation program.

IX

Pharmaceutical Management and Aid for Brain Health

This section is not intended to make you a doctor or to encourage you to demand that you be placed on nootropics, the pharmaceutical term for medications that influence the brain positively.

Pharmaceutical management is an important component of the brain preservation program, especially for people who are just beginning to lose their working memory by forgetting little things like addresses, phone numbers and names of friends and family they used to know.

Nootropics are most effective when used early in the process of brain function decline. They are best used under the supervision of a qualified medical doctor or health care provider conversant with their use.

There are very many nootropics in use, but I will limit my discussion to a few, just to give you some idea about your options in this area.

Dopamine and Deprenyl

Recall, that I mentioned that dopamine was one of the four major neurotransmitters (brain chemicals) when we discussed norepinephrine earlier, the other two being acetyl choline and seratonin.

As people get older, they tend to lose muscle coordination and tremble a little. This is because their dopamine supply is low.

You see, dopamine is the NT for motion and normal muscle control and action. Everybody knows about a major motion disorder called Parkinson's Syndrome. This disorder is caused by dopamine deficiency in some important parts of the brain.

According to some expert researchers on aging and diseases of the brain, after age 40 years people begin to lose ten to thirteen percent of the dopamine they used to have at the peak of their youth every decade until about the age of eighty years when they have less than fifty percent of what they used to have.

As you probably have observed, most of the elders by this age already have some form of trembling in their movements, especially hand movement.

Parkinsonism, however, does not occur unless a person happens to have accelerated dopamine loss and their level is thirty percent or less than it used to be at the peak of their youth.

Some famous people of our time with Parkinson's Syndrome include Mohammed Ali, the former heavyweight boxer; Janet Reno, a USA Attorney General; and The Holy Father, Pope John Paul II.

Dopamine deficiency is not only important because of its role in Parkinsonism and the so-called "essential tremors of aging;" it is also involved in maintaining our working memory. It is dopamine that helps you remember the items on the grocery list you forgot on your table as you left your home to go grocery shopping.

Your normal sex drive and some aspects of your body's immunity are also mediated by dopamine.

With so much of the quality of your life ranging on dopamine, can you really afford not to do something to keep your dopamine levels in the optimal functional levels?

Deprenyl

We have discussed diet and nutritional management stress management, physical and mental exercises and life-style changes that can help to preserve your brain health.

However, if you find yourself slipping despite these efforts, you may need to see your doctor for some pharmaceutical assistance (nootropics).

Deprenyl is one very widely used nootropic. The Europeans have been using deprenyl for decades with excellent results. Some American physicians have started to learn more about it and are beginning to prescribe it. Chances are that over the years more and more people will be using deprenyl as part of their brain preservation program.

The major effect of deprenyl is that it helps the body to build higher levels of dopamine so that the brain does not get depleted of dopamine.

Deprenyl helps you to recover your working memory so that you can remember your grocery list and telephone numbers again. And oh, what a relief that is!

Deprenyl helps you clear that "foggy" head that makes you less confident of your facts. It will help you remember very clearly where you left your car key and go for it.

Deprenyl helps decrease the tremors that low dopamine had induced. This is best if you started to use the medication early in your tremulous disorder.

Experts who know how to use deprenyl would usually start you at very low dose and go up slowly depending on your presenting condition. You could be started with as little as one milligram once or twice a week and taken to as high as 5 to 10 mg daily if you already have Alzheimer's.

The bonus that comes from deprenyl therapy include improvement of any depression you may have, elevation of your mood, increased energy and of course increased sexual desire.

My take on deprenyl is that you should line yourself up with a sexual partner first. I am not too worried about your heart, because if you are already practicing all we have listed in the brain preservation program, your heart will not only be ready for sexual action, but would be jumping for joy at the thought.

By the way, a cardiac exercise stress test is not out of place if you have any doubts about your sexual rush.

The good news is that deprenyl is not like Viagra. It is for both sexes and it is very safe. It is not yet FDA approved in the USA, but Europeans know the asset they have in deprenyl.

Aricept

Aricept is a pharmaceutical agents approved for the treatment and management of mild to moderate Alzheimer's disease.

The neurotransmitter acetyl choline (ACh), which as we discussed, is involved in Alzheimer's, is metabolized (broken down) by the enzyme acetyl cholinestarase. When you have a limited amount of ACh, for whatever reason, and that limited quantity is broken down too quickly, the signs of Alzheimer's become worse.

Aricept is designed to inhibit (restrain) acetyi cholinesterase from breaking down the precious ACh.

Unfortunately, its effect may lessen as the disease progresses, and there is no evidence that aricept alters the course of the underlying dementing process.

It is generally well tolerated in the recommended dosage of 5mg or 10mg per day, but there may be some adverse reactions including nausea, diarrhea, insomnia, vomiting, muscle cramps, fatigue and anorexia (loss of appetite).

People with peptic ulcer disease or those on NSAID (Non-Seroidal Anti-Inflammatory Drugs) pain medication have to be cautious because of the potential for internal bleeding.

DHEA

DHEA stands for de-hydro-epi-androesterone. It is technically a natural supplement and therefore not patentable. But I am including it here as part of pharmaceutical management (nootropic) because it is a form of steroid hormone.

DHEA is a precursor to the formation of the steroid hormones including cortisol, estrogen and testosterone.

It is produced by the adrenal glands but is seven times more concentrated in the brain, where it does most of its work than in the rest of the body.

While DHEA is reputed to impact the rest of the body by improving immunity, normalizing blood sugar, relieving arthritis and chronic fatigue syndrome among other benefits, its effect on the brain interests us in our Brain Preservation Program.

DHEA is said to act as a growth factor in the brain by influencing the neurons to grow more interconnecting fingers (dendrites) so that the communication function of the brain is accelerated.

DHEA also controls that brain intoxicating chemical, cortisol. When DHEA is high, cortisol is low and vice versa.

DHEA can, therefore, be used as a nootropic to lower cortisol levels in chronic stress.

While you can buy DHEA over the counter, it is not advisable to do so without medical supervision, first, because DHEA is a hormone and should be handled like other hormone replacement protocols. This means that your blood level of DHEA, known as DHEA-Sulfate, should be measured before you start DHEA use.

Second, while your DHEA is being replaced, the doctor would have to do periodic blood monitoring to make sure that you are titrated to the optimal level for you.

The doctor would also have to look out for prostate cancer in men by measuring the PSA (prostate-specific antigen) because DHEA can make prostatic cancer worse.

Your liver function studies will also have to be monitored by the doctor if you are on DHEA. So, you can see why DHEA is a nootropic and not just a supplement.

Once your blood tests are in order and you do take DHEA, you will begin to enjoy a qualitatively improved sense of well-being and improved cognition which so many users report.

There is more to DHEA and other nootropics, but this is all we are going to discuss in this section.

The message in this segment is to let you know that you have a wide variety of options in the pharmaceutical management for your brain preservation program.

X

Herbal Management for Brain Preservation

Herbs are natural products usually of plant origin that are reputed to have medicinal or healthy effects in the body.

Most herbs are regarded as tonics, meaning that they help to tune the body up the way you tune the engine of your car.

In the management of brain health, herbs are not intended to wake Lazarus from the dead but to prevent an aging brain from lapsing into degeneration.

Herbs are best as preventive agents, although some herbs, like ginkgo biloba are reported to have the ability to help the aging brain recover some lost cognitive function.

The list of herbs that are supposed to be helpful for brain health is almost infinite. But for our purposes, we are going to discuss only a few of them now. The idea once again is to let you know some of your options.

You should note, however, that all herbs are not created equal. The potency, taste, and efficacy of a given herbal product depend on many variables such as the quality of soil on which it is grown, the amount of sunlight or rain that it received, the cultivation method and even the duration of growth.

Other variables include the method of harvest, preservation, processing and packaging.

Because of these factors, the source of your herbal products is important and when possible, standardization is important.

Green Tea

Teas are a common drink for most people. There is an infinite variety that people drink for various reasons such as stimulation, taste, relaxation, sleep and healing.

Green tea is included in the brain health and brain preservation program, because besides being a powerful antioxidant which fights degeneration by strengthening immunity, it contains flavonoids and caffeine.

The flavanoids, like aspirin, help to prevent blood from clotting, and so helpful in preventing some forms of strokes that are caused by blood clots in the brain.

The caffeine in green tea helps to improve mental alertness, concentration and cognition.

Finally, by helping the liver detoxify the body, green tea helps to rid the brain of toxins that would otherwise becloud it. Green tea can therefore help in dealing with your "foggy" head if taken in moderation—one to two servings per day.

Ginseng

Gingseng is an important herb for brain health because it helps to balance the body's response to stress.

It improves the physical and mental stamina so that we can tolerate stress better.

But most important of all for brain health, ginseng prevents the adrenal glands from producing excess cortisol, that toxic brain chemical that fries the brain in chronic stress. If you get a good source of gingseng, 750mg to 1500 mg daily will be enough to meet your needs.

But like all brain health tonics, gingseng is best taken under the supervision of a competent health care provider.

Ginkgo Biloba

Ginkgo biloba is a world-famous herb reputed as a brain tonic.

It improves the blood circulation to the brain and by so doing improves the availability of oxygen, sugar and other brain healthy nutrients to the brain.

This augmented nutrient and energy supply to the brain improves the brain functions of alertness, attention span, memory and cognition.

Many people report that ginkgo relieves their migraine headache and helps them to remember again.

While ginkgo might help people with mild memory loss regain some of their functions, ginkgo is best used in brain health for preventive intervention.

Ginkgo is safe, but because it improves blood circulation by interfering with one of the blood clotting agents, called the Platelet Activating Factor, excessive use of ginkgo can cause abnormal bleeding.

Do not take aspirin on your own if you are taking ginkgo. And if you are on waferin or other blood thinners, check with your doctor before you take ginkgo biloba.

A dose of 90mg to 160 mg in two or three divided doses is usually adequate.

Lecithin

Recall that of the four major Neurotransmitters (NT), we have discussed norepinepherine and dopamine.

Acetyl choline is the third NT important for normal healthy brain function.

When acetyl choline is low, a person cannot form new memory and cannot gain access to the pre- existing memory.

Acetyl choline is grossly deficient in Alzheimer's disease.

Lecithin is an important source of phosphatidyl choline, a chemical necessary for the production of acetyl choline.

Lecithin, therefore, is important in improving and preventing the loss of cognitive functions of the brain.

Lecithin can be easily ingested in the form of soy lecithin that can be bought as an over-the-counter preparation.

It has no known toxicity, and you can take 1500 mg soy lecithin one to three times daily as part of your brain health protocol.

In addition to protecting your brain from deterioration, you might even get more creative, as some people claim they have become with lecithin.

This is all we are going to say about herbal management in your brain preservation program. As you already know, there are lots of references at the end of this book that you may find useful if you are interested in learning more.

We shall now examine the seventh component of our brain preservation program, Family Love.

XI

Family Love

A popular song by Tina Turner asks, "What's Love got to do with it?" For your brain health and brain preservation program, the reply is "Everything."

We are born into families not just because that is what the genetic code demands but because the family has a role to play in making us human.

It is the family, biologic or adopted, that molds and shapes us physically, mentally, emotionally and spiritually.

Family is so impactful in our character and behavior formation that if a child is brought up by a family of monkeys, he behaves like monkey, and if he is brought up by gorillas, he will behave like gorilla.

What is Family Love?

Family love is caring and sharing with one another in a biologic or adopted family system without the expectation of reward.

Family love is the first glue that keeps functional society together for the good of all its members.

The absence of this "glue" makes the fabric of society fall apart.

Failure to Thrive Syndrome

Observations in the 1930s and 1940s and medical research in the years that followed demonstrated amply that if a child is given all the food and nutrition he needed, but is left abandoned or isolated in a crib or a cage, he will fail to thrive.

In other words, neglected and ignored children do not thrive as normal children do.

To thrive, a child needs love and nurturing. He needs to be picked up, held close to the body, hugged, told he is loved and wanted and made happy in general.

When a child receives these physical outward signs of family love he is happy, filled with laughter, and becomes self confident. Family love encourages a child to be adventurous and to explore his environment fearlessly.

It makes him feel safe.

On the other hand, absence of family love makes it difficult for the child to thrive, fills him with sadness, makes him timid and afraid, and lacking in self confidence.

In place of happiness, he is filled with tears.

He does not feel safe and sometimes becomes paranoid.

Through life every one needs family love to thrive and bring out the best in him.

Unfortunately, many times in our mid life, when we are strong and healthy we get so preoccupied with the immediate goals of achieving success and dealing with the daily demands of life, that we forget the importance of family love.

Or we may take it too much for granted and forget to nurture it, to our detriment later in life.

It is this detriment that has resulted in the current modern trend of isolating the elderly in old people's homes. Society rationalizes this physical, mental, emotional and social isolation of the elders as "good care."

Unfortunately, isolating the elderly in nursing homes achieves the exact opposite of good care; it only helps to put them in the mode of failure to thrive.

In this unhappy mode they begin to regress. They lose the self confidence they used to have, become timid and afraid, sad, frustrated and depressed.

In fact, it would seem that some of the symptoms so-called senile dementia may be, in part, symptoms of regression. The loss of mental function may be due to failure to thrive that in turn resulted from diminished stimulation and nurturing of elders by family members.

Lack of Family Love

Lack of family love is stressful. Failure to thrive is a stress response to isolation and loneliness.

Several experiments in the Caribbean islands in the mid 1980s showed that salivary cortisol levels in abandoned children were six to eight times higher than in normal controls living with their biologic or adoptive families.

You may recall from our earlier discussions that cortisol is toxic to the brain in chronic stress and is responsible for some of the symptoms of senile dementia and Alzheimer's disease.

Similarly, it has been noted that mean cortisol levels in the nursing home population is generally higher than in elders living at home with their families and loved ones. This can mean several things, but the one thing we are certain of is that brain damage by excessive cortisol is more likely to be accelerated in nursing homes than at home.

A good brain health and preservation program encourages you to stay in tune with family love, to keep the chain link of child to parent to grandparent unbroken through out life.

THE MESSAGE: Do not be too busy to care for family and to show that you care.

With few exceptions, if you are there for your child and parents, and if the grandparents are there for the grandchildren, as we will discuss later in this book, you are less likely to end up abandoned and isolated in a nursing home unless unfortunately, you happen to have a disorder that is unmanageable at home where family love nurtures.

I do not want to leave the impression that nursing homes are not good for care of the elders. Rather, I wish to state that home care and family love is better for preserving your brain health.

And you should plan your aging with home living and family love as your preference.

XII

Aging is a Process

Aging is a process. You do not just wake up one morning and find that you are old. Aging happens gradually, almost imperceptibly, one day at a time.

Aging is something you are certain to achieve if you live long enough.

Advanced age is a desirable status to attain. It is so desirable that almost every culture prays for aging and wisdom as trophies of a life lived well.

When you are blessed at birth, you are blessed with long life. People who die before the eighth or ninth decade of life are said to have suffered premature death.

Science, technology and medicine struggle to raise human longevity. They want to extend your life to 120 or more years so that you can truly enjoy your harvest and wisdom years.

While some people grumble their way into and through old age, the majority of people enjoy leaving "childish things" behind for the more esoteric and philosophic "things of age."

Since aging is the law of life, the challenge is not whether you advance in chronological age but how gracefully and healthily you do it, in order that you can continue to retain your mental faculties enough to endow the succeeding generation with your knowledge and wisdom.

Development Comes in Stages, Aging in Pauses

From conception to death we are constantly developing through various stages of life.

Before birth we go from the embryo stage to the fetus stage. We enter the world in the baby stage and then become children. As part of the continuum we go through the pre-teen or pre-puberty stage and then graduate into teenagers and enter the puberty stage.

As we go into our twenties we enter the young adult stage of life and by age thirty we are fully in the adult stage of life.

When age forty comes knocking, we are said to be in the middle stage of life. Some people say that life begins at forty, and I am inclined to agree with that truism. We shall visit the implication of that statement later in this book.

Meanwhile, by age fifty, we are at the maturity stage of life. Age sixty is the advisory or consultant stage of our life.

At seventy we enter the revered stage of the elders. At eighty we are in the senior citizen stage of our journey.

By age ninety we are in the beyond reproach stage of life and if we are lucky enough to make a hundred years, we would have arrived at the celebration stage of life.

Every single stage we pass is a new and peculiar stage of our life as we have not been that age before and will never return to that age again.

The peculiarities of each stage adds to our knowledge and wisdom bag that only we can access and share with others.

The practice of lumping people above the age of 40 or 50 or 60 or 70 into the category of "old" is not appropriate because the stages are as distinct as age one is from 10, and 10 is from 20, or 20 from 30.

The knowledge and experiences of each stage is unique and individually and collectively empowering and enriching.

Aging has to be understood and viewed differently from what many people are currently doing.

XIII

The Pauses of Our Life

Menopause

Menopause is the most famous "pause" associated with aging in women.

Unfortunately, because of the deeply embedded cultural attitude of viewing women's issues as unimportant or outright negative, menopause has acquired some myths around it, especially in western cultures which make social jokes of women who are conspicuously menopausal.

For example, the vaso-vagal instability (hot flashes) that accompany the decrease in the female hormone, estrogen, and which occurs in about two thirds of the women undergoing menopause, provides a vivid excuse for the perpetuation of the myth that menopausal women are crazy or emotionally unstable. Some even call menopausal women witches.

How else could they have explained the behavior of these women, who one minute are happy, comfortable and easy to get along with, and the next minute are flushed red like boiled lobster? Then for no clear reason, they start stripping off their clothes and screaming: "This place is hot! This place is hot!"

Take another situation of a menopausal woman, who before menopause was always happy to have sexual intercourse with her husband and who said she could hardly wait for the children to grow up and leave home so that she and her husband would have a second honeymoon.

Then menopause arrives, and she suddenly loses interest. She even tells her husband not to lie too close to her because she is soaking wet with sweat and can hardly bear to have the bed sheets touch her body at night because it makes her feel like worms are crawling under her skin.

And then her mood swings back again and she feels she could tolerate some sexual contact. She makes some effort but finds it is rather uncomfortable. The vagina is dry. Going for K-Y gel is a chore. She opts to let the whole issue drop and catch a good sleep.

Andropause

"For crying out loud! What do you do with a woman?" the bewildered husband asks as he is left with an erection he had just coaxed from Viagra. He does not find the situation funny.

He, too, is going through his own "pause," called andropause. His erections are not coming as often as they used to come, nor are they lasting as long. This is a strain for him because his male ego is also tied to his ability to unladen his groin of its fullness.

There is tension in the house. The battle of the sexes has become the battle of the pauses.

Brain Pause

Dr. Braverman, of the PATH Medical Group of New York, is an advocate of the pause model of aging. He says that "aging occurs throughout the entire body and that it begins in the brain with electropause."

The brain in a sense is the pace setter for the body. It sends out electrical signals which affect the neurotransmitters and influence the response and behavior of the rest of the body.

The positive electrical brain wave at 300 milliseconds (ms) is called P300. Beginning from age 20 years, this P300 is said to decrease at the rate of about 10ms per decade. This means that by age 70, the P300 will be 50 points less or 250ms.

If the P300 drops too fast, a person develops senile dementia. And if the drop is further accelerated so that the P300 is 220ms or less, the person has Alzheimer's.

Soon after electropause, according to Dr. Braverman, psychopause of the mind with personality changes as measured by clinical indices follows.

Then there comes pineal pause of the pineal gland in the brain, and this is measured by decline of melatonin.

Thyropause of the thyroid gland with decline of thyroid hormone levels and calcitonin comes next and so on until about twenty other body organ systems have paused as shown in Table 1.

Understanding these pauses means that instead of saying some one is crazy or possessed, we can intervene intelligently. With knowledge of the "pauses" in the aging process we can prevent degeneration or loss of function by reversing or controlling the effects of the "pauses" before they become unbearable or irreversible.

We can, for example, intervene in the distress of the menopausal woman by giving her natural or synthetic hormone replacement therapy to compensate for the estrogen deficiency that is causing her distress.

And we can also help the andro-"paused" husband with his Viagra dependency syndrome. He can also be saved the expense of the cost of Viagra and the anxiety about a possible Viagra-precipitated heart attack. He, too, can be given his own natural or synthetic testosterone hormone replacement therapy, with medical supervision, of course.

Understanding the "pause model of aging" is a win-win situation.

Table 1

PAUSE	ORGAN	AGING INDICATOR
Electropause	Brain	Loss of 10ms/decade after age 20
Psychopause	Mind	Personality changes as measured by clinical indices
Pineal pause	Pineal gland	Decline in Melatonin
Thyropause	Thyroid	Decline in thyroid levels and calitonin
Parathyropause	Parathyroid	Decline in parathormone
Thymopause	Thymus	Glandular shrinkage
Adrenopause	Adrenals	Decline in DHEA
Nephropause	Kidneys	decline in erythropoietin level
Somatopause	Liver-pancreas	Decline in growth hormone
Gastropause	GI tract	Malasorption of vital nutrients
Andropause	Testes	Decline in testosterone
Menopause	Ovaries	Decline in estrogen, progesterone, testosterone
Vasculopause	Blood vessels	Hardening and "rusting" of blood vessels
Osteopause	Bones	Decrease in density from malabsorption of calcium
Insulopause	Pancreas	Alteration of glucose tolerance and GH levels
Dermatopause	Skin	Loss of collagen, poor synthesis of Vitamin D
Pituitarypause	Pituitary gland	Loss of multiple hormone feedback loops
Uropause	Prostate gland	Incontinence, atrophy, enlargement, infections
Genatopause	All cells	Alteration in DNA, base pair damage

Reprinted with permission from PATH Medical Group of New York.

XIV

Love, Sex and Aging

This section might be debriefing time for some people because I am going to state categorically that "love is not sex and sex is not love."

It is important that parents get this right and teach their children, especially their girls, that sex is not love and love is not sex.

The confusion of these two issues is responsible for a lot of unhappiness between couples.

Love is a spiritual principle and condition.

Sex is a physical action in an electrically charged physiology.

Love is nurturing and caring for self, others, animate and inanimate substances.

Sex involves satisfying psycho physiological need. It is like hunger for food, or thirst for water. When the need is physically satisfied there is temporary relief until another time.

Love is an open system, sex a closed system.

Sex often has a selfish emotion attached to it. Sex wants to possess. "I have sex with you, so you belong to me. Because you have sex with me, I belong to you."

Love, on the other hand, seeks to give and liberate. Love seeks the freedom of the beloved, not its bondage.

Love is self sacrificing. It is a spiritual principle that is filled with joy the more it empties itself.

This is where a lot of women and some men get confused. When love empties itself, we are talking about its spiritual self, not its physical self.

Sex empties the physical self and leaves one physically exhausted.

People who confuse love with sex, especially women, run themselves ragged to please their partners. They wash, clean, mop, dry, bake, cook, fry and do all kinds of other good things and top it off with sex hoping to find love. What they find instead is physical exhaustion and emotional drainage.

This is because they are looking for the living among the dead.

Sex is good, and it has its own fine place as low-grade physical combat with chemical pleasures attached. It is also designed for procreation and should be enjoyed and utilized appropriately.

Sometimes sex and love can be shared by two people as husband and wife, but it happens less often than we wish. Otherwise, the divorce rate would not be over 60 percent.

Traditional societies and early western civilizations understand these two entities well enough to base family traditions on arranged marriage, which is simple expediency and a physical arrangement.

Recurrent association of sex and love by Hollywood movies has created the illusion that the two are one and the same. Unfortunately, they are not.

In one of Oprah Winfery's shows in February 2000 she reported that forty million American women admitted they were having sex "out of duty."

When you are doing something because it is a duty, there is no freedom and no choice. To be duty bound is to be in bondage to that to which you are bound.

We do not have statistics on men, but I suspect that a lot of men are having sex either because of a sense of duty or the need to relieve themselves of their physical urges rather than as an act of love.

I do not want to be misunderstood. Sex can be an act of love, if it is utilized as a sharing and caring vehicle, but it does not have to be, and often is not.

Eating can also be an act of love, but most of the time we do not eat because of love; we eat because we are hungry.

Now let's take a good look at love itself before we examine the beautiful place of sex in aging.

What is Love?

Love is a state of being, a state of living.

There is only One Love with two components. The first component is love for God, and the second is love for everything else.

Love for God, as explained in my essay, "Understanding Spirituality: It's like the Computer," is known simply as obedience to God's commands, if you believe in God.

Love for everything else begins with awareness of the existence of the object of love. People who do not love themselves, for example, consider their own existence null and void. Not validated. They have annihilated themselves psychologically and so cannot care for or nurture what does not exist—themselves.

Self respect is a state of love.

Friendship is a state of love.

Marriage is a state of love.

Family is a state of love.

Acts and attitudes that reflect the presence of love include kindness, empathy, generosity, humility, understanding, tolerance, and forgiveness.

Where Does Love Come From?

Initially, I did not understand why the love for God is obedience, while the love for every other thing was a state of being.

Then I realized that God does not need the endowment of kindness, empathy, generosity, understanding and tolerance from me. I am the one who needs these endowments. To receive them before I can share them with others, I must go to God who is Love, the State of Love, and the Source of Love personified.

Here is a good analogy.

Suppose you have a bucket of water, with a faucet at its bottom and a lid on top. Think of the bucket as your body, and the water inside as the love you contain.

When the faucet and lid are closed you have nothing but a bucket full of water. Nothing is coming in, and nothing is leaving.

In that state you cannot water the flowers, relieve others of their thirst, or wash clothes, because to perform these functions, your faucet has to be open.

However, your faucet is controlled by a mechanism that automatically opens the lid of the bucket the moment the faucet discharges some water.

The bucket is positioned in such a way that the lid is in the direct path of a large reservoir of water that automatically fills the bucket as soon as it discharges water. This mechanism ensures that your bucket is always filled with water no matter how wide you open your faucet and no matter how much water is discharged for daily activities.

This illustration is the same as saying, "The more you give, the more you receive."

Your ability to provide water is limited only by the size of your bucket.

Love Disconnect

Suppose you decide to move your bucket away from the water source?

What would happen if you opened the faucet and there was no source of water to refill it?

The bucket will be drained out of water and become empty.

An empty bucket cannot provide drinking water, washing water, bathing water, garden watering water and so on.

So, what would you do if you do not want your bucket to become empty? Shut the faucet, of course.

But when you shut the faucet, the bucket still cannot provide water, so it becomes technically useless for those specific purposes.

To become functional again, you have to return the bucket to its source of water.

Note that your removal of the bucket from the source of water does not destroy the bucket; it just made it less functional and less useful.

Similarly, separating yourself from the source of love, does not destroy or kill you physically, but like the empty bucket your lack of love, makes you less functional and helpful to people and things around you.

Only One Love

There is only one love. As in the analogy above, there is only one supply of water.

Obedience to God is the exactly the same act of love as caring for and sharing with others.

Since God is Love and the source of love, to receive love, you have to be in line with the source of love, equivalent to positioning the bucket directly under the water source.

This direct positioning is what we call obedience.

If the bucket is not filled with water from the source, it cannot dispense water. The bucket does not manufacture water. Similarly, we do not manufacture love, and if we are not filled with love from the source, we cannot dispense love.

But once the bucket is filled, if it does not dispense its water, it cannot be refilled. It must give to receive, empty itself to be filled.

This is a fundamental spiritual law.

And we did say that love is a spiritual principle. In fact, it is one of the three spiritual principles that guide our lives. The other two are Faith and Hope.

"Faith, Hope and Love, and the greatest of these is love."

Understanding love and learning how to give, share and receive it is the wisdom of aging.

E-Language for Love

Put in e-language, obedience is the mode in which we download instructions from the source of love. It is after that, that we can, print out, dispense our love (empty ourselves of) kindness, generosity, tolerance, forgiveness and other acts of love.

Obedience to God's commands is the download mode of love; the acts of love are the hard copy printouts.

I did tell you in the book, *Understanding Spirituality: It's Like the Computer,* that e-language is the modern language for understanding spirituality and our life.

Love is no exception.

Now, let's go to the fun part: Sex and Aging.

XV

Sex and Aging

Sex and aging is the fun part because we are humans.

Now that we know that love is not sex and sex is not love, let us "ru uuum mmble!"

Well, not quite.

The big problem with sex is that it is a closed system.

An act in which two people repeatedly confront one another in search of pleasure can only produce so many highs and "fireworks" before it becomes boring or merely tolerated for the sake of peace.

As I mentioned earlier, forty million American women, in a survey reported by the Oprah Winfrey show in February 2000, say that they engage in sexual activities, "out of duty." That fact should tell us that we are not doing it right,

If we were doing sexual activities properly, why would so many people be dissatisfied with it?

The first answer is that it is not the sex act itself that is incorrect, but the expectations from the act.

The act itself promises us the possibility of only one of two outcomes. The first is the possibility of temporary pleasure. The second is the possibility of conception and procreation.

And if you fall in the category that I am writing this book for, conception is no longer an option. So sex is purely for pleasure.

Why is the pleasure elusive or so hung up in all kinds of distractions?

Sex is Not for Power Struggle

The first incorrect expectation of sex is using it to control our partner.

Let me be explicit in saying that a lot of sexual activity among the aging is probably outside marriage because many in this group may have lost their spouses through death, divorce, abandonment and other ways.

My message is about consenting, aging adults who may or may not be married.

When you go to rumble with the intent of controlling the other person, the body language and emotions transmit the truth of your intentions to your partner so that instead of pleasure, there is contradiction and tension.

Sex is Not an Anti-Depressant

If you approach your partner with the idea that sexual activity would lift you out of depression, you make a mistake.

In many instances you depress your partner's mood and end up more depressed and fighting. If you are depressed, work out your depression first before sex.

Sex is Not Your Toilet

If you approach sex as a relief of physical pressures in your groin, your partner will pick up the signal and resent you.

Where there is resentment, pleasure disappears.

Sex Should Not be Bound by Law

It is human nature to be rebellious.

"Laws are made for humans and not humans for laws."

Laws are made to be broken. It should not be surprising, therefore, that once we take a vow that we are bound to someone, the next thing is to look for an excuse to break the vow.

People have been known to break their vows on their wedding night.

There is something about vows that take our freedom away. And we want our freedom back.

"Let your Yes be Yes and your No be No," Christ advised us.

Imposing an oath is a waste of time. Look at the statistics—a 60 percent divorce rate.

Don't demand that your sex partner commit to you. If you are good, he or she will be faithful.

Do not forget to practice safe sex. Old people can catch bad bugs from sex too.

Enjoy Sex as Dance

As you advance in age, if you are a man, most likely you have some degree of impotency and do not have the acrobatic endurance you used to have. Go slowly on sex like a slow dance.

If you do that, you might get to meet and know the woman you have been taking for granted for so long and begin to see her as a full human entity instead of a mere sexual tool.

And if you are a woman, as you advance in age, you may find that you have turned off sex because of your experiences as a younger woman. Now that you are not part of the forty million young American women, you do not need to feel the necessity for the "duty of it." Your vagina is dry most of the time anyway, and you get urinary tract infections just from the thought of sex. So you abandon the whole show.

Once in a while you feel the urge for intimacy, but you are worried that your partner, who barely holds on to his own erection, might just satisfy himself and leave you unsatisfied and angry with yourself for ever thinking that he, who did not come through when he was younger, would come through now.

The message is; "Don't lose hope. He, too, is getting more mature and is learning to wait."

The woman should also approach sex as a slow dance. Just take it slowly, talk as you used to do when you slow danced Enjoy the comfort and warmth of your partner and worry less about your dryness because if you both slow dance long enough, you will both ultimately "get it," and the quality is so much more full and satisfying than anything you ever had in your younger years.

Trust me. I got this information from "reliable sources."

Don't just enjoy sex as slow dancing. Put on some music, your favorites.

Be friends first

You must be friends with your sexual partner. You must share common grounds and interests, especially as you get older and sex becomes more of a head than a groin project

You need friendship to laugh and joke, tease one another and play pranks.

You need friendship to discuss important issues and to plan.

You need friendship for quality time and stress reduction.

When friendship is in place, sex becomes a part of sharing that friendship.

If you are not friends with your spouse or sexual partner, when either of you is unable to "perform," you have nothing else to talk about or share, and disappointment and resentment take over.

Sex, the Symphony of Age

Sex is a low-grade combat contact sport, full of fun and excitement

For the aging it must become a well choreographed dance. Beautiful to dance to in harmony. Discordant when out of tune

With age, sex provides the pleasures of matured wine. Deep, rich, velvet.

When played as music sex replaces the Rock 'n' Roll of Youth with the Symphony of Age.

Sex is for the Living

Sex is for the living, not the dead.

You know there is no sex in heaven because Jesus told us so.

So if you like sex and you have the right motives, enjoy it like a good glass of wine. Sip at it, savor it and enjoy it

Then hang on to its flavor and glow or float all week long. You've got time.

Surely your partner is worth savoring and if you do not think so, don't waste time having sex with him or her.

If you do not like wine, you do not drink it

The goal of sex as you get older is to enjoy it. If you do not enjoy its complexity, you must honor and respect yourself enough to say, "No."

XVI

Drug Abuse and Aging

When we think of drug abuse, we often think about the youth.

But with time youth become the aging. And like everything else, we carry our baggage from youth to old age.

If you abused drugs as a young person and have not been rehabilitated or seriously handicapped by your abuse, chances are that as you get older, you will continue to abuse drugs.

Drug abuse in the aging is not a popular topic because people are afraid of being offensive. And rightly so. But it is a subject we must discuss in a book about wisdom of aging.

Our purpose is not to condemn drug abuse in adults and elderly but to acknowledge it and then go beyond it.

If you abuse drugs and other substances, recall how you started this behavior.

If you enjoy the behavior and your health and purse are not compromised by it, there is no reason to encourage you to change the behavior.

If on the other hand, you do not like the habit or behavior but find yourself unable to stop, then you may wish to make a list of all the advantages and disadvantages of drug or substance abuse to you.

After making the list, you may wish to search within yourself for the reason why you do it.

Chances are that you will come up with the answer that you are trying to "feel good," "fill a void inside you," or "do something because you are bored with yourself."

Chances are also you will find that the drug abuse does not really fill that void because when the effects of the drug wears off, you still return to your own empty self.

The reason is that drug abuse is a symptom not the disease.

The real disease is the reason you feel empty.

You feel void or empty because you have not validated your spirit.

When you validate your own spirit, your own "I Am," you link it up to, or anchor it to the Universal Spirit, which is God. Then you feel complete.

This is when the emptiness or void is filled.

The good news is that when this void is filled, you have no further need for drugs. Drug abuse is actually a spiritual defect with physical symptomatology.

Drug or substance abuse is a dependency problem. You depend on the drug or substance to rescue you from whatever is bothering you.

But drugs do not have the power to rescue you. They are only chemicals that delude you temporarily.

Simple logic tells you that if you depend on drugs you cannot depend on anything else, including God. This is so, because the very word "depend" means "resting your weight or purpose on" the thing you are depending on.

This explains why it is almost impossible to stop drug abuse without a "rescue squad" in the form of counselling and support system.

Counseling succeeds when it helps you to find yourself by validating your spirit within you.

If you are getting older and drug abuse continues to plague you, you should seek counselling or read books and practice mind-body exercises that may help you validate your spirit

You may find that my little day-by-day book, *Meeting and Knowing Yourself,* will help you do this.

A validated spirit liberates you from drugs and substances, so that you are set free to really enjoy your life and advancement in age, in sound physical, mental and emotional condition.

XVII

Alcohol Abuse in Aging

What I said about drug abuse is also valid for alcohol abuse. The only difference is that alcohol abuse does not have the social and legal stigmata that drug abuse carries.

The dependency symptoms of alcohol abuse come from the same place as the dependency symptoms of drug abuse and the solution is the same.

This is not to say that there is no place for moderate alcohol use in the life of people as they get older. There is plenty of space for alcohol in the aging population. We only caution against the abuse or excessive use of alcohol.

And even for small to moderate use of alcohol, we note that alcohol is a drug and can affect some of the medications that you may be using for your heart, arthritis or blood pressure.

It may also be a good idea to check with your doctor or pharmacist about medication interaction with alcohol for all your medications and supplements, regardless of whether they are prescription or over the counter.

Alcohol and drug abuse are bad for you and make things worse as you get older. Besides the damage these abuses can do to your general health, they destroy your brain cells at very accelerated pace and may push you into early dementia or Alzheimer's disease.

Your brain is your most important asset especially as you get older because it makes it possible for you to use the wisdom you have acquired over your life time. If your brain fails, your wisdom fails. You must be protective of your brain as we discussed earlier.

XVIII

Quality of Your Aging is Your Choice

The choices we make to a large extent determine who we become. We are always in the state of "becoming" all through our life.

Children become adolescents who become adults, who become parents, grandparents and mentors, elders and guardians.

Our parents make the initial choices for us. They choose which baby sitters look after us, which kindergarten or elementary school we go to.

By high school or adolescent years, we are considered old enough to make some of the choices for ourselves. We choose what extracurricular activities we participate in, what clothes we wear, which college we wish to go to, and which trade or profession to pursue—with advice from parents, teachers or counsellors.

Later on we choose if we wish to marry or not to marry. We choose our spouses and our careers.

For every choice we make there is a consequence.

If, for example, we opt to go to Harvard instead of State College, our teachers will be different. Our classmates, friends and environment will be different from what it would have been if we had chosen differently.

The choices we make determine the next set of choices that we would have.

For example, if we choose not to go to college, then we will not have the option of becoming doctors or lawyers because these professions need a college education.

If we choose to drop out of high school, we pretty much know that the possibility of us being stuck in low paying jobs is very high, unless we happen to have other talents which present us with other choices.

Choices must always be made with an eye on the future.

XIX

Every Choice is Important

Every choice you make is important.

There are no major choices and no minor choices as far as your future is concerned.

Some people consider marriage choices and investment choices such as buying or bidding on a house as major choices.

But these choices are no more important than choosing to say "Good morning" to your spouse or significant other on waking up, brushing your teeth, washing your clothes, going to school or showing up at a soccer game.

Every choice, no matter how universal or how personal it may be, is important.

As much as we would like to blame our unpleasant experiences on others or on the system, most of what happens to us is the harvest of choices we made earlier on.

Take for example, a seventy-year-old man suffering with cancer or liver pain in the hospital. Even if he had inherited the genes for the cancer or disease, which he could do nothing about, the expression of the gene was determined by the choices he made in his younger years. Choices like eating poorly, smoking two packs a day of cigarettes for years, consuming large quantities of alcohol or abusing drugs repeatedly over the years.

The consequences of our choices sometimes come so much later that we forget that we made the choices that led us to the harvest of distress.

Some may seek exceptions to the rule of consequences but unfortunately, there are none because Nature does not lie.

The sun never rises in the west.

Some may say, What about the poor old woman dying from lung cancer who never smoked a day in her life?

What about where she lived and worked, the water she drank and the foods she ate?

If it were possible to play back every minute of her life, step by step, we would most likely find where she made the choices that ultimately resulted in her current situation.

There are no accidents.

You are where you are based on the choices you made previously.

The good thing about choice is that you can unchoose. You can opt out of previous choices by correcting your errors and choosing differently.

For example, if you choose to eat high calorie meals and become fat because of it, you can unchoose high calorie meals by eating fewer calories, and you will become less fat

If you choose to consume meals that clog your heart vessels, you can also unchoose those meals and with time your heart vessels will become unclogged.

The general rule is that choices that produce rapid results can also be reversed rapidly. And choices that take a long time to produce consequences need a long time to reverse once you unchoose them.

The bad news is that many of the people who are neglected and abandoned in nursing homes have earlier on made choices that led them there. Sounds callous, but it is true. It is the law of nature.

The message is—choose wisely. Every choice has a consequence, and every choice matters.

So now that you know that your choices create your future, you can choose to plan your aging years to be happy, contented, healthy, pain free and wise.

XX

Plan your Aging for Happiness

Common sense and expediency require that you plan your aging.

"You should not just stand there and wait for decay. You should Do Something!"

The two forces that keep the balance of life are the force of rejuvenation and the force of decay.

You have a choice as to which force you pitch the tent of your life with. The choice you make determines your future and how you age.

Some people in their twenties wake up each day complaining that they are getting old, because they will soon be 30 years old.

Others in their thirties complain that life will end when they hit age 40.

Still others pretend they do not have birthdays because they think that the additional candle would burn them out.

Well, I have good news for you. It's celebration time. Enjoy your aging. It's a new beginning. Your aging begins your wisdom years. The years for which function you were born.

Childhood to Adulthood

When you were a child your parents or guardian planned what kindergarten, elementary or primary school you attended.

They decided what you ate, what you wore, where you slept and a host of others things.

From high school or adolescence onward, you began to take some control of your life, planning what college to attend or what career you wished to spend the prime of your life pursuing.

You also planned other things such as what to eat or drink, what to wear, where to visit for vacation or sight seeing, who to go out with or "hang out" with.

Later on, you planned who to marry, where to live, when to have children; if at all. If you did not plan your life, it would be chaotic. And a chaotic life is stressful.

Life is a Journey

Life is a long pleasant journey that takes your lifetime, which is currently 80 years and may take up to 120 years if healthy lifestyle, medicine and technology have their way.

No one goes on a journey without planning it, unless it was an emergency trip.

A traveler usually has a purpose for his journey—business, vacation or personal. He usually seeks for some information about his destination, if he did not already know about it.

Next, he plans how to get there: air, land or water. Group trip, small company, or alone.

He considers what he will need on the way to his destination: clothes, food, water and other items.

Travelers plan their journeys because they wish to have trouble free journeys if they can.

If you traveled and had a rough journey, you would arrive your destination tired and exhausted. But if you had a smooth journey, you would arrive happy and in positive anticipation of the purpose of your journey.

Life is a journey, and aging is only a segment of the journey.

You do not arrive at aging overnight.

You would have traveled from birth to childhood to adolescence, adulthood and maturity. You would have had time—10, 20, 30, 40, 50, 60, 70 or even 80 years as the case may be to plan your journey.

You should therefore not be surprised or upset on arriving at the age of wisdom. In fact, you should be happy, excited and ready to enjoy the endowment of your new status.

You should be elated to share, and not regret the stories of your beautiful and unique life's journey; with its fantastic moments filled with fun and laughter. Yes, there have been occasional hitches here and there, but that is what makes the arrival triumphant.

So, how do we plan the aging segment of this awesome journey?

XXI

Have a Vision

You should have a vision of your wisdom years. You should be able to close your eyes and see yourself in your old age.

Are you happy? Are you surrounded by loved ones? Are you comfortable? Living where you wish to live? Eating what you wish to eat? Engaged in the activities you enjoy? Free of fear and undue anxiety? Healthy, content, sharing your knowledge and wisdom with your children, grandchildren, and those you mentor?

If this is your vision, keep it and live into it.

If, however, your vision of yourself shows a person who is sad, depressed, weepy, lonely, incapacitated, weak, unhappy, anxious, hungry, poor and abandoned, then you need to change the picture.

And if your vision is blank, you better fill it up with something swell, or else all kinds of debris will fall in there for you.

As we said earlier, your vision creates your future.

Your vision of your future is your prophecy. But you can choose to unchoose that future and create a different and happier one. You have the power within you to be whatever you wish to be at any age, if you so choose.

As we said at the beginning of this book, you must conquer all your fears in order to live out your dreams. And your dreams are actually your visions of tomorrow of yourself.

When you were younger, you called them dreams; as you get older, you call them visions.

You need to have a vision of your wisdom years because as a traveler on the road called life, your vision is your destination.

Make it fabulous for your own sake.

XXII

Getting to Your Vision

Getting to your vision, your destination as created by you, is equivalent to the routes and transportation systems used for a trip and the nourishment you had on the way.

The five basic requirements for your journey to your destination or vision, are air, water, food, shelter and nurturing.

The joy or lack thereof in your journey is affected by the quality of these five items that you package to take along with you.

The choices you make on your way in this journey to your vision is your lifestyle.

Air

You need fresh, clean air to keep you alive and provide you with the optimum oxygen you need for your lungs, heart, brain and every cell in your body.

If you live in a polluted environment, whether you caused the pollution or not, the quality of air you breathe will impact the wellness of your lungs, heart, brain and everything else in your body.

Also you can further compromise the quality of oxygen you breathe in, if your lifestyle choices include cigarettes or any other substance, smoking, working with dusts and fumes or inhaling dangerous drugs.

If living with a respirator or chronic attachment to an oxygen tank is not part of your vision, you have to make the appropriate choices of excluding them in order to materialize your future.

If, however, you are already struggling with compromised air to your lungs, you may wish to see your doctor and follow the most rigorous modern medical advice to improve your condition.

It might also be a good contribution to the wisdom of mankind if you would become a profound advocate for the necessary changes by government or industry to ensure that necessary precautions are taken so that people who have to earn a living in air-compromised environments are safeguarded from their negative consequences.

Water

Water is an important item that impacts how you get to your vision—that is, arrive at your destination.

You need clean water for a healthy life.

You need clean water for drinking, bathing, doing your laundry, cooking, washing, and a whole host of activities of daily life.

In addition, clean unpolluted water is necessary for the health of plants and animals.

If you drink unclean, contaminated or polluted water, you endanger your health with infectious diseases, vomiting and diarrheal disorders. You can also get hepatitis and a whole host of cancerous disorders.

If your vision of your wisdom years do not include chronic disorders like cancer caused by water pollution, you should ensure that you drink clean filtered water and that you avoid exposing yourself to waterborne diseases.

Again as in the case of polluted air, if you are already a victim of the disorders caused by unclean, contaminated or polluted water, you should see your doctor and vigorously pursue whatever you have to do to restore your health.

Again you could become an advocate for clean safe water, using the wisdom of your experience to help others avoid the health consequences of unclean water.

Food

You have most likely heard the statement, "You are what you eat." You need healthy foods as we discussed earlier on to build a healthy body. You should also know that "Junk foods make your body a junk body."

Exercise caution in what you put into your mouth. If you choose to load up your body with refined sugar, excessive salt and preservatives that mortify foods; blood clogging fats and empty calories that blow your body up and cause your bones to degenerate, then you are voting for a vision of you with multiple bypass heart surgery, possible strokes and paralysis, osteoarthritis and other nutritionally facilitated degenerative disorders.

You may also be voting for high blood pressure, kidney disease and a host of cancers of the digestive system and the other organs.

Your food as an adult is your choice. And the fastest food is not necessarily the best. Eat with a purpose of good health in your wisdom years as a vision.

Shelter

You need a reasonably decent shelter appropriate to the climate and environment where you live. It should not be too hot and not too cold. You should not be exposed to extremes of temperatures for good health.

You need clean, well-ventilated housing. You need space for your routine daily activities and for relaxation also.

Some people prefer spacious living quarters while others prefer smaller more compact spaces. Whatever your preference, put it in your vision.

If institutional living, surrounded by strangers and unfriendly care givers, is not in your vision of your wisdom years, then do not place it there by making the wrong choices.

Plan the resources you are going to need for what will make your old age living arrangements comfortable and acceptable for you.

Discuss these with your loved ones when you are still young and vigorous. Do not wait until you are on the verge of being institutionalized before you talk about these issues.

Your living arrangement in your wisdom years is probably the most important and most conspicuous evidence of your vision of your future.

You have the power to place yourself comfortably in your vision and the time to do so is now.

Nurturing

As we have discussed in detail in this book, nurturing is very important for your total health; mental, emotional, physical and spiritual.

In getting to your vision that is your wisdom years' destination; you need to be nurtured yourself.

You have to be kind to yourself because you are unique and wonderful and not because you wish to impress onlookers.

You must say nice things to yourself. “I am beautiful.” “I am handsome.” “What a gift from God I am!” “I look terrific.” “I love my hair.” Look at those eyes.” “Look at the muscles.” “Whaaoo!”

“I am kind, I am gentle, I am considerate. I work hard, I love people.”

Do not depreciate yourself by saying bad things to yourself, such as, “I am too fat. Look at that ugly belly. I am getting too old. I am no good. I am a pain.”

Don’t say negative things about yourself because your words create you.

Your thoughts are the possibilities, but they have no effect unless they are spoken, created by your words or concreted by your action or behavior.

Put differently, your wisdom years are put into motion by what you think, while what you say creates it, and what you do manifests it.

You must nurture yourself also by doing nice things for yourself from time to time. Send yourself flowers, buy presents for yourself.

Groom yourself well. Go to the spa or sauna Get a massage. Relax, sing, pray, appreciate yourself.

How can you envision being nurtured by others if you do not nurture yourself? How can you complain that your significant other, parents or children did not send you flowers or gifts if you did not do the same for yourself?

How can you say you are abandoned by others, when you abandon yourself?

Nurture yourself by reading good books, listening to good music and speeches, and watching good movies and television programs.

And please, don't ask me to define "good;" you know what is good for you.

Junk begets junk.

From what you nurture yourself with, you will nurture others

This is all we are going to say about nurturing for now. Next, let us examine where the money you will spend in your wisdom years will come from.

XXIII

Where is the Money?

You most likely have heard the financial companies advertising for people to plan their retirement by putting some of their money away in savings accounts, mutual funds, bonds and various investment portfolios.

You probably have some pension money or "nest egg" stored away for your wisdom years.

Yet, the experts and some government authorities repeatedly say that the very old and the very young, at the two ends of the spectrum of human life span, are the poorest members of the population.

You were probably one of the "authorities" in your younger days who made this kind of statement.

If you have worked most of your adult life and have put away some money for retirement, how is it that you can still be classified as relatively poor in your wisdom years?

The answer is, first of all, that your pension is usually less than your last full pay check. You are not receiving the same amount of money you were getting before retirement. That means that retirement gives you a pay cut.

Next, inflation and the annual rise in the cost of living eat into your now limited pension so that your money does not go as far as it used to go.

Finally, because your physically aging body requires more attention and care, you are now probably spending more money for your preventive and curative health management than you did in your younger years.

At the end of the day, it appears that indeed, your wisdom years would be part of your financially poorest years. But is it unavoidable?

My position, is that you need not be poor if you include some or all of the ideas we are going to discuss now.

Nest Egg or Retirement Income for How Long?

If you retire at age 65, and had planned to put away enough money to last you till the end of your life calculated as 80 years but you live to age 85 years or more, then you have at least five years of abject poverty waiting for you at the end of your wisdom years.

That does not make you look very wise to the young.

If halfway through your anticipated fifteen years of pension you realized you were still healthy and that your chances of exceeding your eighty-year life expectancy was good, what can you do? Spend less money for food, vitamins, medications and other things that have kept you healthy? Worry about your potential poverty until cortisol kicks in and starts eating your brain?

This would not make you look wise, either.

Perhaps the first thing to do, since you are living in this third millennium, is to anticipate that you will at least celebrate your one hundredth birthday in good health, and 120 years is not far fetched.

Your vision of your aging should therefore be far enough to save you undue anxieties in your luxurious years of wisdom.

Now, I ask, "If our chances of living to age one hundred years is very high, at this point, in our collective human journey, what are we doing retiring at age sixty-five?"

How do you plan to spend thirty-five years in retirement? Decay? Be productive?

XXIV

Do Not Retire: Begin a Passion

I tell a story to my executive class when we discuss stress and retirement.

I tell them that a lucky person should volunteer to receive everything he could possibly wish for from me. I offer the person all the money he wishes, all the food, drinks, clothing, jewelry, cars, houses and any thing else he wants, provided he did just one thing for me.

At this point every one wants to know what I want, but I will not tell them until one of them commits himself to giving me the one thing I ask for in exchange for all the goodies of life.

When I get a volunteer, I say, "Please, sit here. That's all I want you to do. Do not go anywhere. As a sign of my love, I will bring everything to you here. I will bring your commode here and bathe you here and..." Before I go any further I hear a chorus of "No! No!"

"Why?" I ask in surprise.

"That's not love!" they tell me. "You want to kill him."

"How can I want to kill him when I am offering him everything he desires.?" I still act surprised.

"Don't you know that if he does not move he will die?" They tell me.

That is exactly the message. If you don't use it, you lose it.

As we discussed earlier in this book, if you do not use your physical body or brain, it will go into atrophy and lose function.

Retirement puts you on the fast track for disuse atrophy of all systems.

You cannot afford to retire, at least not until you are about to transit this earth to another realm. You need to work, no matter how minimally, because you need to be physically and mentally active to be healthy.

Suppose your company's employment policy offers you an irresistible retirement package after so many years of work, or after a certain age, and you feel you have to comply. You may cease that particular employment, but you must not stop being busy. This is the time to begin a passion.

What is a Passion?

A passion is something you have always loved but have never really had the time to give it appropriate attention.

You may have a passion for photography but never had the time to practice photography because you were too busy with your career as a plumber or tailor or whatever.

You may have a passion for animals, birds, fish, the forest or wildlife.

You may have a passion for arts, crafts, sculpting, painting, drawing, designing and so on.

I have a passion for music, especially piano music. I always have a piano in my house, but I still cannot play the piano. I have every intention of being a concert piano player—at least a little concert player—some day.

Who knows, I may even cut a CD of my wisdom age piano music and may even have it published on the internet!

Practicing piano and taking piano lessons is in my vision of my wisdom years. The brain cannot weaken or the body tire when there are still challenges to meet.

Everyone has a passion. Note your passion and put it into your vision of your wisdom years, so that when you terminate the career of your youth, you can begin the passion of your life.

When you pursue your passion, you elevate it, and it elevates you.

For you your passion will become fun and productivity its harvest And it does not even feel like work!

Your passion often adds to your material wealth, because you are committed to it, because you love it, and because you do it so well.

Your passion should be the basis for your third career.

You can envision your passion at any age, but if you have not already done so, the best time to do it is now.

The act of envisioning yourself being involved in your passion begins your post retirement or "wisdom age" career. This is super insurance for you, because it will ensure you do not just wait around for physical and mental decay.

You will be Doing Something!

XXV

Do Not Retire: Decrease Your Work Day and Week

You may feel that you have already put in enough work hours for a lifetime of even 120 years and simply do not wish to work any more after your retirement.

Or you may not feel fit enough to continue as vigorously as you used to.

Your post retirement years may be an opportunely to do something new and different from what you have done to that point. It may be a time to work for yourself, work for others, or to pursue your passion at a calculated pace.

Working for less hours, say three to five hours a day and for fewer days, say two to four days a week, may give you all the pep you need for a whole new life experience in your wisdom years.

A decreased work day and week will make fewer physical demands on you and give you time for more leisure and fun while ensuring that you do not suffer the consequences of the disuse of your physical body and brain.

The time you save from working only part of a day or week can now be invested in enriching your spiritual self, sharing your wisdom with every one and raising the future generation.

Take a Sabbatical

You may wish to begin your wisdom years with a sabbatical.

When I was approaching my fiftieth birthday I decided to take a sabbatical to do something completely unrelated to my profession. My friends asked me how I could go on sabbatical when I was self employed and was not a teacher.

The perception at that time, among my friends, was that a sabbatical, was for university professors only.

I thought differently.

"I am my own boss," I said, "and I am giving myself a sabbatical."

I took the sabbatical and what a change and renewal of life I found!

This book is one of the incredible results of my taking a sabbatical at age fifty.

And it just keeps getting better.

Taking a sabbatical will not only refresh you but may give you ideas that you will need for another 50 years to give you great satisfaction.

You do not have to take sabbatical only once in a life time. You can take one every ten or twenty years, or any time you need a prolonged change.

These days you don't even have to travel physically from one place to the other for a sabbatical. You can take your sabbatical in cyber space.

This brings me to the topic of cyber space and your wisdom years.

XXVI

Cyber Space: A Wisdom Age Medium

Internet technology has created a world so exciting that one may need several lifetimes to explore, navigate and enjoy it all.

You do not have to be young and strong to surf the net. You do not need to be super smart. You do not have to be rich. And you do not even have to be articulate to surf the net.

In fact, you do not need a fabulous state of presence of mind to surf the net. Even if you have some age-associated dementia, you can surf the net.

Surfing the net is intellectually stimulating and will strengthen your brain the more often you surf.

I have an idea to visit every continent in the world and every country in it in the cyber virtual world.

Can you imagine the excitement of visiting one country on planet earth each day on the internet? You would be learning about different people, languages, customs and traditions. You would visit various historic sites and enjoying the peculiar geography and natural beauty of each country. You might even make a few friends while visiting.

Can you imagine visiting all the museums in the world without having to travel to all of them.

What about visiting major libraries in the world without ever leaving your home? Reading all the books you wish on the net? Visiting craft shows, listening to music, watching movies, buying, selling and doing countless other things on the net.

The internet provides you with so many options that sitting in a nursing home peeping hopelessly out of the window should not be one of them.

And by the way, those who own and run nursing homes should provide Cyber Cafes for their residents (an idea of my sister Claire), who are willing and able to use them. They can also be used for mind rehabilitation programs.]

Create Your Own Web Site

There is room for everyone on the net.

If you are alive, there is space for you on Earth. And if you have space on earth, you have space in cyber.

Use your own web page to tell the universe about yourself. Say good things about yourself, provided they are true.

Cyber space is particularly suited for the aging population as a tool to teach their wisdom.

Physical strength is not required in cyber space. The shape and size of your body is irrelevant.

Cyberspace is not affected by your race, color or creed.

Even if you do not know how to create your own web page, countless people and programs can help you put one together. What are you waiting for?

Flaunt What You Have (Wisdom)

Youth has strength and energy; competing with them for those is futile.

Adults have employment, financial resources, power and clout going for them. Struggling to recapture any of these from them is defeatist.

Since wisdom is your domain as you age and youths are not competing with you for it, flaunt it. Spread your wisdom in cyber space.

And while you are at it, enjoy your new self. Be happy and grateful for who you are.

Stop complaining about your lost youth and vigor.

Celebrate the knowledge and wisdom in your aging.

XXVII

There is Wisdom in Aging

There is wisdom in creation.
Aging is part of the creative energy cycle.
It is not an accident.
It is not a punishment.

Everything ages.

Human beings age.

Animals age.

Plants age.

Cars age.

Houses age.

Your clothes age.

Everything ages.

There is wisdom in aging because aging is a process of natural recycling in obedience to the law of conservation of energy.

Every scientist knows that the total energy in the universe is fixed, but in a dynamic flux between its potential and kinetic (dynamic or motion) states.

Total energy can never increase or decrease.

So, in accordance with the law of conservation of energy, when dynamic energy (force of creation or rejuvenation) increases, the potential energy, (force of rest or dormancy) decreases and vice versa.

Quick or very fast changes in moving from the dynamic or kinetic state of energy to the potential or dormant state of energy or vice versa is physically expressed as violence.

A volcanic eruption is an example of sudden change in energy states. The explosion of an atomic bomb is another extreme example of violence.

A ripe mango falling off the mango tree, on the other hand, is a less violent example. However, the end result is the same: a changed energy state.

Aging is a Change in Energy States

Aging is yet another example of the physical expression of the changes in energy states. It is simply a more gentle and slowed-down change from the dynamic or kinetic physical state of being to the resting or potential energy state of being.

The ultimate goal of the universal energy system is to maintain balance. This is what the scientists call enthalpy or homeostasis.

The most efficient way to maintain this balance is by returning every matter, (visible or dark matter) to its elemental composition.

"Dust to dust Ashes to ashes."

Youth and Aging are Two Sides of the Same Energy Coin

Aging is a controlled energy transformation from dynamic to resting.

Because sudden changes like volcanic eruptions are violent and disruptive of other steady states around it, nature, in its creative and resource management wisdom, designed a gentle and gradual breakdown and recycling system called aging to limit the number of violent changes associated with energy state transitions.

This gentle recycling system is built into every cell in the body. This is why we have enzymes, hormones, vitamins and cofactors. They are placed within our body metabolism to keep us from exploding from our own atomic energy reactors during our kinetic (anabolic and catabolic) growth dominant stage of life.

After adulthood and reproductive stages, they are withdrawn.

To re-cycle our borrowed matter (our body), in compliance with the law of conservation of energy, the gradual withdrawal of the activities of the enzymes, hormones, vitamins and cofactors, eventually turn down the furnace of our metabolism until the last embers go off peacefully and we return “elements to elements.”

Aging is a Kind and Considerate Process for Energy Transformation

Aging is, therefore, a kind and considerate way of maintaining energy balance and order in a universe in which violence (sudden changes in energy states) would otherwise be the status quo.

Mars and other planets where energy exchanges are more violent illustrate what can happen to physical life as we know it when violence is the status quo.

“Where is the wisdom in controlled energy transition?” you ask.

Answer: "The wisdom is in the opportunity to experience physical life, as we know it, on planet Earth."

If there were no energy transition control mechanism, no one would live long enough to age. In fact no one would survive the birthing process because the energy for transition from womb to the atmosphere is so great that one would explode at birth.

And if any one made it through birth, he would burn into ashes and disappear into the air within days because one needs so much energy exchange to build one's body from the elements in the milk, food, water, and air one consumes to build one's physical body.

In fact, without this controlled energy transfer, you would not have been conceived because there would have been no surviving woman to birth you and no surviving man to father you.

No birthing, no youth; no youth, no aging.

Youth and aging are the two sides of the same energy coin.

So now that we know that both youth and aging are in compliance with the natural law of conservation of energy, how do we extract the best lessons and experiences of our slow, kind and gentle energy recycling (a.k.a. aging) to enrich humanity and endow future generations?

By teaching the youth.

XXVIII

Teach the Youth Your Wisdom

Because the aging process takes so many years to extinguish the burning embers of our lives, the elders in general have enough time to teach the young people from their repertoire of wisdom and knowledge.

There is a consequence for the elders, if they do not teach the youth.

In a Bible story, Hophni and Phinehas, the two sons of the chief priest, Eli, and priests themselves, were frivolous and disrespectful in following God's instructions. They demanded and took the fat portions of animal sacrifices that were supposed to go to God in the smoke of burnt offerings.

> If the man said to him (Eli's sons), "Let the fat be burned off first, and then take what you want,"... (Eli's sons) would then answer, "No, hand it over now; if you don't, I'll take it by force." (1 Samuel 2:17)

Unfortunately, their father behaved like many a modern parent does these days. He barely gave them a slap on the wrist.

> Now Eli, who was very old, heard about everything his sons were doing to all Israel and how they slept with the women who served at the entrance to the Tent of Meeting. So he said to them, 'Why do you do such things? I hear from all the people about these wicked deeds of yours. No, my sons; it is not a good report

> that I hear spreading among the Lord's people. (1 Samuel 2:22-24)

Since every choice has a consequence attached to it, when judgment day came to Eli's house, it was total devastation.

> "Why do you scorn my sacrifice and offering that I prescribed for my dwelling?" God asked Eli. "Why do you honor your sons more than me...?
>
> "Those who honor me I will honor but those who despise me will be disdained. The time will come when I will cut short your strength and the strength of your father's house, so that there will not be an old man in your family line. Every one of you that I do not cut off from my altar will be spared only to blind your eyes with tears and to grieve your heart, and all your descendants will die in the prime of life." (1 Samuel 2:29-33).

When I asked my little girl why depriving the Eli family of "old men" was a punishment, she said because the "Old people are supposed to provide wisdom and authority for the family."

"Aha!" I said to myself.

The youth perceive the elders as their source of wisdom and authority. When the elders, like Eli, abdicate their responsibility for one excuse or another, they are still liable for the actions of their children. Even grown children.

Eli's two sons were grown men and priests in their own right. Still the elders, in this case their old father, owed them direction and rectitude.

The message here is that teaching and guiding the youth is not an option, it is an obligation for the elders, failure of which results in grave consequences.

Many twenty-first century elders act like Eli. "What do you expect me to do?" they ask. "My children are not kids. They are grown men and women."

"Do better than Eli," the Creator demands, "or face the harvest."

With the judgment on Eli's house saying, "(his) descendants will die in the prime of life," it becomes clear that aging is a privilege, not a right.

The privilege of aging, of having the gradual and gentle energy transition from one state to another, discussed above, was being withdrawn from Eli's family in favor of the more violent energy transfer because he had not trained his children well.

There is consequence for not teaching the youth.

If any generation of elders do not teach the youth as they should, they will not have peace in their old age because the "sons of Eli" (youth) will disturb their peace in Columbine and similar places.

So, for your individual and everyone's collective well being and peace in old age, you must teach the youth.

XXIX

What Do You Teach the Youth?

Everything.

Children are born without knowledge, experience or wisdom, as far as we know. They have to learn every thing.

The trick in teaching the youth is to begin while they are still babies, but it is never too late to teach anybody at any age.

If you are a first time parent, guardian or mentor, this is an opportunity to do everything right the first time.

If you are a grandparent, grand uncle or aunt, or a second generation mentor, this is a second chance to get it right.

And if you are a great grandparent, guardian or mentor, this will be your third chance to get it perfect.

If you have the privilege of beginning with a newborn baby, you should begin by telling this little person that he or she is the best, the most beautiful, the most wonderful, the most precious one in all the world, the one who will achieve the greatest in life and bring the greatest happiness and joy to the world.

These fine words cost nothing. You do not need money or resources to program your baby for goodness.

The first thing to teach a child is cleanliness.

Cleanliness

Start teaching children about cleanliness at the very earliest age, possibly at six months and definitely by eighteen months.

Teach children how to clean and pick up after themselves, no matter how sloppily. Of course you should still pick up and clean up after them, but they must be made to put in their own little effort first. In this way they learn that their effort is required and appreciated by the adults and the family.

They also enjoy it.

As children get older, you must insist that they learn how to bathe daily, wear clean clothes, and learn to wash their own clothes even if you have to re-wash the same pieces after them.

Teach them how to keep their environment clean, participate in gardening and in yard work. Early practice of cleanliness eventually make cleanliness second nature.

The health benefits of cleanliness is known to all. And the saying that cleanliness is next to godliness will become a bonus.

Obedience

If you think obedience is out of date, then the law is out of date.

Society expects everyone to obey the law. The foundation for law-abiding citizenry is laid in the obedience they learned at home as children.

Sometimes parents and grandparents leave training of their children in obedience to school teachers only, or to religious leaders alone. They may be afraid their children would resent them or perhaps they do not care enough to make the required effort. The result is that their children tend to make more preventable major mistakes.

There is always a sad consequence waiting in the future for disobedience.

Children must obey their parents and lawful elders. To do differently, would be to recreate the story of Eli's sons as we discussed earlier in this book.

Truancy at school is a sign of disobedience of school rules and regulations and a signal of potential difficulties with the law in the future for the child.

The final social consequence of lack of obedience is a breakdown of law and order in the community and resulting negative impact on harmonious and peaceful living.

Gratitude and Appreciation

One of the first signs of the decline of a civilization is ingratitude.

When people stop saying "Thank you" and "please," they are headed for a sad fall.

It is not old-fashioned to say "Thank you."

Good manners never go out of fashion.

Because it is a proud heart that does not recognize appreciation and greediness that leads to ingratitude, you must teach children to be grateful and appreciative of other people's efforts on their behalf, no matter how small the effort is.

If you give a child a piece of candy, he should say "Thank you," and if you wipe his runny nose, he should also say "Thank you." If he does not, teach him how to say "Thank you" and explain to him why gratitude and appreciation are important.

Understanding

Understanding is an attribute that makes for harmony in the family and the workplace, among friends and in society at large.

You must teach the children to be understanding of other people's points of view.

Understanding does not mean agreeing with whatever the subject is. It simply means taking a moment to view a given issue from a perspective that is different from yours.

Understanding allows the spirit of tolerance to thrive.

A good way to teach understanding is to have the children learn the art of debating. This allows them to look at the pros and cons of any given issue dispassionately.

Understanding, ultimately, becomes the foundation of wisdom.

Listening

Children should be taught to listen.

The impetuousness of youth make children "Me Centered."

When today's youth were infants, they cried for attention, and adults responded by feeding them, changing their diapers, picking them up, rocking them or providing them the desired comfort. This is perfectly appropriate.

But the children also learned that the louder they cry, the more urgently their needs are attended to.

However, as they grow old enough to talk and express themselves, they should be taught to listen also.

They must learn to hear what is being said to them. Hearing is important.

Many times elders talk to children who are not deaf, but do not hear because they have not been taught to listen and to hear.

Listening includes taking a moment to let the words or sounds register in the brain, thinking about what is said before responding.

One way to teach a child to listen and hear is to ask him, "Do you hear what I am saying? Do you understand what I said? Please repeat what I said in your own words."

This appears tedious at the beginning, but it will save everyone a lot of grief later on in life.

You have probably heard wives complain, "He does not hear what I say. He does not listen to me."

Does it surprise any one that divorce rates are high? Too many spouses have not learned to listen to one another.

Another way to teach a child to listen is never to shout above the child's voice. Some parents make the mistake of shouting and screaming in the hope the child will "hear" them. It does not work that way.

The statement, "When you want to capture someone's attention, WHISPER," seems most apt for teaching children to listen and hear.

Humility

Teach your children humility. It will earn them favor before God and man.

Pride and arrogance are fruits of self destruction.

Pride leads to conceit and disobedience.

"Pride is always about falsehood," making things bigger than they really are. Exaggeration.

"Humility is always about truth," knowing more but claiming less.

I learned this from an EWTN TV commentary during Pope John Paul II's visit to the Holy Land for Jubilee 2000.

Humility earns respect and leads to understanding and harmony.

Harmony leads to peace.

And peace is necessary for progress.

When you teach your children, grandchildren or wards how to be humble, you will sleep better.

Saying, "I am Sorry"

No human being is without mistake.

This means that from time to time, children will make mistakes that they are responsible for.

You must teach children to say "I am sorry" when they have erred, instead of arguing or pretending to be faultless.

The legal and corporate systems that encourage people not to accept liability are morally wrong.

They teach the people to "gain the whole world and suffer the loss of their own souls."

Everyone should take responsibility for their choices and actions.

Saying, "I am sorry" is a gentle and considerate way of taking responsibility for one's errors.

Ethics

Ethics must be taught.

You have to teach children to be honest and true in everything they do and to treat everyone fairly.

Cheating and lying should never be acceptable, no matter how convenient.

By being fair and firm with your children, grandchildren and wards, their recollection of you later in their lives will always be that of gratitude and joy in having had you as a mentor.

I recall when I was about nine years old, a tomboy, always in for adventure and excitement, I had had a fallout with a neighbor's child, and the parents reported me to my mother.

When judgment time came, I was told to recount my own side of the dispute.

As I started to talk, I was stammering because I wanted to tilt the account in my favor, but before I could do any damage, my mother very calmly but firmly said to me, "Don't even think of it. Even if you killed a person, and I came and asked you if the allegations against you were true, I expect you to say 'Yes.' At which point I would go on my knees on your behalf and ask for mercy."

At this point, my story froze in my mouth.

I have never forgotten that lesson and all through my life, you can never get me to put my name on anything unless I understand it to be true.

Naturally, I have demanded the same standard of my own children.

Generosity

You must teach children generosity. They must learn to give and to share.

As we said earlier, children are born with the physical survival instinct of self centeredness.

"Me! Me!

"Give Me! Give Me!

"I want! I want.

The child cries when he wants food, cries when he wants water, cries when he is wet and wants to be cleaned, and cries when he wants to sleep.

If you ignore a child's cry, it will cry until it is exhausted.

Take a toddler to the shop and he wants to buy all the candies or toys. He wants this, and he wants that, and unless you teach him the limits he will not stop.

Generosity does not come naturally.

Children have to be taught to be generous.

Love and Respect

I have written extensively about love elsewhere in this book. The message at this point is that children should be loved and then taught how to love and respect God, their parents, teachers, elders, guardians, and mentors.

Children should also be taught to respect themselves and their peers. Respect begets respect and gives value to one's sense of self.

The preceding teaching is for all children and youth. We wish now to take a look at specific teaching for the youth.

XXX

Gender-Specific Teaching for Youth

If the elders in their wisdom years choose to see peace in their community, they should try to transfer to the children some gender specific tips for harmonious living.

Gender Specific Affirmations for Girls

One of the biggest problems for girls is low self esteem or lack of self-confidence, which force them into living less fulfilling lives or into subjecting themselves to mental and physical abuse.

Every elder in his or her wisdom should decide what is appropriate for the specific environment The statements included herein are suggestions only.

Little girls should learn to assert themselves without being overbearing.

Teach them to say the following, and be prepared to explain to them why you are teaching them these affirmations because they will ask you for the meaning of what you are teaching them.

I am somebody.

I am important.

I have a specific reason for my life.

I am not a property of anybody—parent, brothers, sisters, friends, husband or any one else.

I am an independent, thriving and responsible person.

I will contribute positively to society.

I will be ethical in all my dealings.

I will be honest and fair to all at all times.

I will be responsible far all my actions and not blame any other person for my mistakes.

I will respect my parents, teachers and elders.

I will respect every human being appropriately.

I will respect God.

I will respect myself at all times.

I will not subject myself to abuse by anyone.

If anyone attempts to abuse me, I will not keep it quiet. I will tell everyone around me—parents, teachers, friends, guardian, religious elders, pastors, priests, rabbis, about my abuser, and I will go to the law to report that person so that no second attempt will ever be made on me.

I will not be used as an object or plaything. I am a human being with a soul.

I will draw the line for self respect. If any one attempts to cross that line, I will say, Stop! And if they do not stop, I will fight for my self respect, within the law.

I will have the best education I can possibly have within my own limits.

My life is a gift from God.

My life is not dependent on any other human being.

I am a winner.

This kind of assertions can go on and on. The point is that children generally do not know their potential because of their age.

When you are a child, everyone is a giant, but by the time you know the difference, your brain has already been imprinted, sometimes with unhappy events.

Assertions help children prepare for the intimidators of life.

Gender-Specific Affirmation for Boys

Boys are the brothers, fathers, grandfathers, uncles, friends, husbands, and sons of girls.

There should be no wars between the boys and the girls. The two should be complementary to each other.

We need boys and girls to make the human family and create universal harmony.

Affirmation for boys is to help them improve their own self esteem also and to be assertive as well without being brutal in spite of their physical strength.

They should be able to say things like this:

> I am a human being.
>
> I am made in the image and likeness of God, but I am not God.
>
> I am a gift to my parents and to myself.
>
> I have a specific mission for my life.
>
> I am a kind and gentle person.
>
> I am an understanding and forgiving person.
>
> I am friendly.

I am a determined person.

I am hard working.

I am honest.

I am sincere.

I take responsibility for my actions.

I respect God.

I respect my parents, teachers and elders.

I respect every one regardless of their race, color or gender.

I am willing to listen to other people's viewpoint.

I am polite.

I am not violent.

I will never hit a girl or woman.

I will not be involved in gang activities.

I will always keep good company to the best of my knowledge.

I am determined to get the best education I can possibly get.

I am helpful to all people in need especially those weaker than me.

My life will be a positive influence on any one that I come across in my life.

Planning for General Life and Marriage

The reality of human life is that we do grow up, get married or share our personal lives with significant others.

The majority of human beings do get married, so we will look briefly at some of the things we should teach our boys and girls to consider as they get older and begin to consider sharing their lives in marriage.

Each person should have a written list of the following:

Things you like

Things you do not like

What makes you happy

What makes you unhappy or sad

What makes you angry

What do you think about money—important, not so important, center of everything?

What do you think about poverty—important, not so important, center of everything? Avoidable, unavoidable, chance, destiny?

If you were rich, how would you manage your wealth? If you were poor, how would you cope?

If you were married and were the rich partner, how would your money be controlled and managed?

If you were the poorer spouse, how would you like your spouse to manage his or her money?

If you were married, what would your attitude toward your spouse's parents and family be?

Would you consider your in-laws part of your family—or intruders?

Would you like to share your husband or wife with them?

What is your attitude to extended family?

What is your idea of a nuclear family—just you, your spouse and children and nobody else?

Do you like to receive visitors?

Do you prefer to be left alone?

Do you think others can help you?

Would you give freely to family members, or would you rather they keep their expectations off your money and resources?

Do you think it is acceptable to hit your spouse or partner, or to be hit by them?

I strongly recommend that as a way of limiting domestic violence, every home should have some sports equipment such as a punching bag, soccer ball, basketball, ping pong table, treadmill, or dumbbells for weight lifting. A punching bag is highly recommended for those who have a tendency to strike out at their spouse or children. It does not take up much space and also helps keep them fit.

The above topics and others you may wish to add should be reviewed at least once a year on New Year's Eve or on your birthday.

Be sure to share this list with the person you hope to marry or share your life with long before you exchange rings.

Better to have him or her go through the same topics you have reviewed and write his or her own responses down, too, so that you can exchange your views and have an open discussion long before there is need for a shouting match in your marital home.

Understanding your matured attitude towards important issues will help you understand your intended life partner's DOS and DON'TS and help to create a more harmonious family life.

XXXI

How to Teach the Youth

Now that we have discussed when and what to teach the youth, we will take a look at how to teach them.

Teaching the youth is a major issue for the aging in their wisdom years, because it is vital to their peaceful transition and the progress and stability of society.

Children are born neutral. They are neither well mannered nor bad mannered at birth.

They are born clean and unadulterated, like VCR tape on which nothing has been recorded. Like the VCR tape, they will record anything that is presented to them and play it back on cue.

The generation of children that follow is a product of their parents' generation. What they exhibit in their behavior is a display of what their parents severally and collectively have recorded in them.

We should not ask, "Where does this generation of youth come from?" because they come from us.

If they are good, respectful, kind, happy, friendly, considerate, caring, modest, empathetic, gentle, humble, truthful, honest and God fearing, we have so planted.

And if they are disrespectful, cruel, unhappy, unfriendly, violent, inconsiderate, selfish, vulgar, unsympathetic, arrogant, proud, boastful, dishonest, untruthful, non-God fearing and ruthless, we have so planted them severally and collectively.

You do not have to be a biologic parent to teach the generation of youth following you. You teach by example. The children learn by seeing, hearing, and feeling. They use all their senses, including smelling and tasting.

When they meet adults at school, work, play, or at a place of worship, they do not say: "This adult is a parent, one I will emulate or copy. This other adult is not a parent, one I will not copy or emulate."

No, children see adults as a group, the same way most adults see the youth as a group. If the adults would not view the youth as a group, a different generation, the question, "Where do these kids come from?" will not arise when a young person(s) commits an atrocity as was the case at Columbine High School in April 1999.

Children learn from the adult generation before them. This means that all the adults have the responsibility to teach the youths.

This is as good a time as any for me to say that every adult, religious or not, should attempt at some point to read the Old Testament of the Bible, at least for its historic perspective about the preceding generations teaching the following generations.

For example, in the book of Judges as Samuel records the beginnings of Israel's defeat in Canaan, the promised land, he said—

> "After that whole generation (that is those that returned from Egypt and settled in Canaan) had been gathered to their fathers, another generation grew up, who knew neither the Lord nor what he had done for Israel." (Judges 2:10)

(I must note that Israel is both a reality of a people and an allegory for all mankind who recognize God as their Father.)

The preceding generation of Israelites (those who inherited the land of Canaan) were so preoccupied with their abundance, successes and daily struggles that they did not take the time to teach the next generation about what the Lord had done for Israel.

In the same way we are too preoccupied with our own material and intellectual abundance, successes, deadlines and daily struggles to remember that teaching the children is part of the insurance policy for the peace and progress of our nation and mankind.

Just as the new generation of Israelites in their "ignorance" of what is right, "did evil in the eyes of the Lord and served Baal," (Judges 2:11), the new generation of our mankind, our children, are doing what is evil in our eyes and in the eyes of God. They are serving Baal in the form of greed, violence, disrespect and sexual abuse of self and partners.'

Unfortunately, they were not well taught by their parents' generation. To our chagrin, the youth are the ones that pay the price.

The ignorant, untaught children of Israel suffered the consequences of their ignorance.

> "In His anger...the Lord handed them over to raiders who plundered them..." (Judges 2:14)

Similarly, the generation of our children, who have not been well taught by us, are paying the price with a high incidence of depression, drug abuse, loveless sexual escapades and suicide.

They are being raided and plundered by soulless technology. They are confused. They are looking for teachers who will teach them right, and that is your job as you get older and wiser.

Teach a Younger Person One Good Thing Each Day

As you get older, make time to teach at least one person younger than you one positive lesson a day. It could be a wise saying from the Bible, or from folk tales, fairy tales, newspapers or magazines.

If you do not live with a younger person, get into some mentoring program or help teach kindergarten or pre-school children.

The opportunity to teach youth abounds, and they are ready to learn.

You may think you are not computer literate and wonder how you can teach modern kids.

But if you reflect for a moment, you will realize you have a lot to teach them.

What about your carpentry and fishing? Crocheting and knitting? Needlework, basket weaving, cloth weaving, banking, gardening, quilt making, hand painting, pottery skills, drawing, singing, dancing, classic piano, guitar playing, playing cards, playing scrabble, playing chess?

While it may be possible to learn about these skills from the computer, the human interactive transfer of knowledge from person to person has a value-added impact that cannot be quantified.

In these transfers you enrich the souls of the next generation and make them divine.

There is no excuse for any adult whose brain is still intact not to teach a younger person every day.

If you do, your own soul will also be enriched.

I recall an incident in which I was on a train ride to New York City with another lady in her 60s.

The seats assigned to us were occupied by two young people about twenty years old. When I told them those were our seats, they scoffed at us and told us to go to the back somewhere to find seats for ourselves.

I found that unacceptable and protested their attitude and behavior.

Meanwhile, the other passengers in the train were anxious to take their own seats and urged us to go and "find another seat." Others were scared that the youths might turn violent if I insisted on what was right and wanted my protest to stop so they could assume the false peace that would hopefully follow.

Since I did not wish to contribute to the temporary chaos any longer than I needed to, I told the two young people, "This is wrong and you know it, and you will pay for it someday."

And then we went to find seats for us.

While it appeared on the surface that the youths had won a temporary victory over their elders, their minds were troubled.

How did I know it?

About twenty minutes into the train ride while my friend and I were in the dining car for some snacks, one of the two youthful "victors" came up to me.

When he had finally caught my attention, he said, "Ma'am, I am very sorry for my behavior. I always make it a point to respect my elders. I don't know what got into me this time..." Before the statement was finished, I said, "You are forgiven," and followed that with a mother's hug.

The joy on the youth's face was ecstatic!

Did the kids learn anything from that encounter? Of course they did and they learned it for life. Did I fail in my teaching duty that day? Of course not.

There is no fear when you teach the truth.

Fear abounds where falsehood is nurtured.

The message, is—

Teach the children

They want to learn

They will learn.

We must teach the children, because if we do not teach them well, with time, "Innocence is lost while Wisdom is out of reach."

I do not recall if this is my quote or someone else's, but it sounds good and I defer to whoever made the first statement, "Innocence is lost," because the VCR tape we started with at birth has been recorded by time.

Too often wisdom is out of reach because the recording is fouled, distorted and so unpleasant to play back!

XXXII

A Good Model for Teaching the Youth

Many classic and professional books that try to teach us parenting skills, family interaction and social skills, but I have found none as sound, concise, comprehensive and enduring as the four chapters of the book of Ruth in the Bible.

You do not have to believe in the Bible to read it, just like you do not have to believe in Shakespeare to read *Macbeth!*

At the very least, you can view the Bible as a great library of knowledge on all the issues of our lives.

I have found that teaching the young people from the book of Ruth opens the door for major discussions on youths, adults, men, women, the old and society at large.

It is a short book about the interactions of a functional family.

The Story

Briefly, the story is about a man called Elimalech, who took his wife Naomi and his two sons, Mahlon and Kilion, to a far away land to settle, because there was famine and suffering in their home town of Bethlehem.

While they were there, Elimalech died and left his wife and two sons behind. The two sons married two local girls, Orpah and Ruth.

Unfortunately both sons died before they could have children.

It had been ten years since Naomi migrated. Having lost her husband and two sons, and learning that the famine in Bethlehem had abated, she decided to return to her people.

Naomi advised her two daughters-in-law to return to their respective families as they were young widows, and their chances of re-marrying would be better among the people where they were known.

Orpah returned to her people after much persuasion from Naomi, but Ruth refused to leave her mother-in-law, opting to return to Bethlehem with her.

Ruth in Bethlehem

When Naomi and Ruth arrived in Bethlehem, Ruth worked for their daily bread by going to the barley fields and picking up the left-over grains (gleaning) after she obtained permission from the field workers.

It turned out that she was gleaning in a field belonging to Boaz, a man of wealth and standing, who happened to belong to the same clan as Elimalech, Ruth's late father-in-law.

When Boaz arrived at his farm, he greeted his harvesters, "Peace be with you." As he greeted them, he noticed a strange woman in his field and asked his foreman who the young woman was.

The foreman told Boaz the woman was Ruth, the foreigner who had returned with Naomi. They also informed Boaz that Ruth was hard working.

> "She went into the field and has worked steadily from morning till now, except for a short rest in the shelter." (Ruth 2:7)

Boaz welcomed Ruth and gave her permission to stay on and glean and to follow his servant girls.

> I have told my men not to touch you. And whenever you are thirsty, go and get a drink from the water jars the men have filled. (Ruth 2:9)

Boaz then commended Ruth for her devotion to Naomi and bravery in leaving her home land to come and "live with people you do not know before." (Ruth 2:11)

The story tells us that Ruth continued to work hard and carried home to her mother-in-law, Naomi, the day's gleaning and whatever extra food she had left over after eating. She also gave Naomi detailed information about her daily activities.

Naomi Teaches Ruth

Naomi, like a concerned and loving mother, did not want Ruth's youth to be wasted.

> My daughter, should I not try to find a home for you, where you will be well and provided for? (Ruth 3:1)

Naomi then instructed Ruth on how to get the attention of Boaz, because as a close relative, according to the Jewish traditions, Boaz was in line to inherit Ruth as a wife.

> "Wash and perfume yourself, and put on your best clothes," Naomi instructed Ruth. "Then go down to the threshing floor." (Boaz will be winnowing barley on the threshing floor.) "Don't let him know you are there until he has finished eating and drinking. When he lies down, note the place where he is lying. Then go and uncover his feet and lie down. He will tell you what to do." (Ruth 3:3-4)

Naomi completed her instructions.

Ruth did what she was told and got Boaz's attention.

A Kinsman-Redeemer for Ruth

Instead of Boaz taking advantage of Ruth by pretending that he was drunk when he woke up to find Ruth at his feet in the night, he behaved like a gentleman with honor and dignity.

> "Although it is true that I am near of kin," Boaz told Ruth, "there is a kinsman-redeemer nearer than I. Stay here for the night, and in the morning, if he wants to redeem, good; let him redeem. But if he is not willing, as surely as the Lord lives I will do it. Lie here until morning." (Ruth 3:12-13)

Boaz followed the protocol for redemption and transfer of property without looking for any shortcuts.

According to the requirements of his culture, he asked the first kinsman redeemer to choose freely if he wanted to buy Elimalech and Naomi's sons' land from Naomi and accept Ruth, the young widow, as well. But the man opted not to buy the land and redeem Ruth, because, he said, "I might endanger my own estate." (Ruth 4:6)

Having refused the offer, the first kinsman-redeemer in the presence of witnesses on both sides, took off his sandals and gave them to Boaz to symbolize the final transfer of all rights to another person.

With this transfer of rights properly accomplished, Boaz said,

> I have also acquired Ruth, the Moabite, Mahlon's widow, as my wife, in order to maintain the name of the dead with their property, so that his name will not disappear from among his family or from the town records. Today, you are my witnesses. (Ruth 4:10)

Ruth Blesses Naomi with a Grandson

Now that Ruth was properly married to him, Boaz fathered her son Obed.

Naomi in her old age is once again fully enriched.

Naomi was so filled with love and hope that the villagers said to Naomi,

> "Your daughter-in-law who loves you and who is better than seven sons, has given him (Obed) birth."

And of Obed, they said to Naomi,

> "He will renew your life and sustain you in your old age."

Naomi, the grandmother, responded by nurturing and caring for the youth and hope of the future.

> Then Naomi took the child, laid him on her lap and cared for him. (Ruth 4:16)

How exciting!

No matter your age, when you nurture a child, he becomes yours and your future. So the villagers said, "Naomi has a son." (Ruth 4:17)

Ultimately, Obed grew up to become the grandfather of King David.

Principles from the Story of Ruth

The story teaches so many vital principles for a happy life, that after reading it to children, I ask them to make a list of the characters of Ruth, Boaz and Naomi.

Here is a summary of the teaching points under each person's name that the children and I have discussed. You may find them helpful, too.

Ruth

Ruth, symbolic of Youth shows—

Fearlessness and Adventurous Spirit

She was willing to go to a foreign land with her mother-in-law, unafraid of the potential dangers that lay ahead.

Endurance

Under the hardship of a young widow, she was willing to start life over and make the best of it.

Commitment

She was committed to her new family and mother-in-law, Naomi.

Devotion

She was devoted to the service of her mother-in-law and her new community.

Hard Work

She worked in the field all day long.

Persistence

She kept struggling to provide for her own needs and the needs of her mother-in-law.

Obedience

She followed the directives of Naomi without argument.

Simplicity

Simple in her desires. Not greedy. Boaz remarked, "You have not run after the younger men, whether rich or poor." (Ruth 3:10)

Openness

She told her mother-in-law all that happened to her in the field. Who gave her gifts and who said kind words to her.

Gratitude

She showed gratitude to Boaz by thanking him politely. "At this she bowed down with her face to the ground." (Ruth 1:10)

Boaz

Boaz, symbolic of Man of Substance, shows—

Humility

He greeted his harvesters, "The Lord be with you" first. He did not stand like an ogre waiting for the harvesters to come and fall prostrate before him.

Open Mindedness

He welcomed Ruth, a foreigner, without constraints.

Kindness

He told his harvesters to "Rather pull out some stalks from the bundles and leave them for her (Ruth) to pick up, and don't rebuke her." (Ruth 2:16)

Of Boaz's kindness, Naomi had said, "He has not stopped showing kindness to the living and the dead." (Ruth 2:20)

Protector

He did not want a stranger to be assaulted in his community. "Stay here with my servant girls—I have told the men not to touch you." (Ruth 2:8-9)

Hard Working

He did not just leave the work to his foreman and his harvesters. "Tonight, he will be winnowing barley on the threshng floor." (Ruth 3:2)

Integrity

Even if he desired Ruth, he did not harass her or take advantage of her, by using "being under the influence of alcohol" as an excuse.

He respected his own honor and dignity. And he respected Ruth's honor and dignity as well.

He followed the due process of redemption before marrying Ruth.

Discretion

Though he had no shameful relations with Ruth, he did not choose to "brag about a young woman chasing him, even unto the threshing floor."

So she lay at his feet until morning, but got up before any one could be recognized. "Don't let it be known that a woman came to the threshing floor." (Ruth 3:14)

Selflessness

He might have been interested in Ruth, but he was willing to be selfless in the cause of what is right by allowing the first kinsman-redeemer to exercise his full right first, even if it meant that he would not get a chance to marry Ruth.

"...If he wants to redeem, good; let him redeem. But if he is not willing, as surely as the Lord lives, I will do it (Ruth 3:13)

Generosity

He knew that Naomi still needed someone to provide for her, so when he gave Ruth some barley, he gave her in excess, so that Ruth could take some to her mother-in-law, Naomi.

"He gave me these six measures of barley, saying Don't go back to your mother-in-law empty handed," Ruth informed Naomi. (Ruth 3:17)

Naomi

Symbolic of the Aging, shows—

Fortitude

Naomi, her husband and two sons had gone to another land to escape physical hunger and hardship, but she returned stripped of all her assets, except for her widowed daughter-in-law, Ruth.

But she bore her trial with fortitude and was determined to go back home to Bethlehem.

Consideration

Naomi was willing to set her two daughters-in-law free, so they could continue with their youthful lives.

She could have held them hostage and used them to fill the void of the loss her husband and two sons, but she chose to give the young women the option to go or not to go with her to Bethlehem.

Farsightedness

Naomi, a single parent head of a household of two, wanted a good future for her daughter-in-law, Ruth, because she knew that she (Naomi) would not always be around for her.

"My daughter, should I not try to find a home for you where you will be well provided for?" (Ruth 3:2)

Wisdom

Naomi used her wisdom to advise Ruth on how to get the attention of Boaz.

She did not attempt to compete with Ruth. She had played the role of "being there" so that Ruth had someone to share her daily experiences with, as she went out daily to earn the bread for the family.

Knowing who you are, and your role at every stage of life, is part of wisdom, and Naomi lived the practicality of wisdom.

Love

Naomi played out the practical role of the aged by caring for and nurturing the next generation of youth, Obed.

Then Naomi took the child, laid him on her lap and cared for him. (Ruth 4:16)

Obed

Symbolic of the Children and Humanity's Future, shows—

Renewal and Sustenance of the Aged

The women of Bethlehem in their collective wisdom told Naomi, "He (Obed) will renew your life and sustain you in your old age." (Ruth 4:15)

The cycle is completed. Naomi though a grandmother and old, is not discarded. She begins to nurture the child who is the future.

This makes her once again like a young woman, and the villagers said, "Naomi has a son!" (Ruth 4:16)

Functional Family

The story of Ruth is the story of a truly functional family and of good choices. Every major character in this story made the right choices.

The consequence of their individual and collective choices, resulted in their individual and collective joy, peace, harmony and abundance.

They all had the opportunity to choose differently. And if they had done so, the results would have been different.

Ruth could have opted to stay behind with her sister-in-law, Orpah.

Naomi could have chosen to use her two daughters- in- law, selfishly as "hostages" to her life of big losses. She could have also chosen to advise Ruth badly and possibly steered her into the life of prostitution for quick money.

Boaz could have chosen to be arrogant and abusive. He could have taken sexual advantage of Ruth before the due process was completed. He could have ignored the whole protocol, because he was rich and powerful and not given the first kinsman-redeemer any options to choose whether he wanted Ruth or not.

The story of Ruth is definitely not the only story that puts the specialized roles of the various age groups into a cohesive interplay of morality, consideration and dignity for all.

You may know or have other books and stories that do the same thing as the Book of Ruth does for teaching cohesive functionality in family and society. Pick them also, if you wish.

The net objective is to find a story that is short and simple enough for young people to read and form a basis for teaching and sharing your wisdom with them.

If you do this, the youth will always remember you with respect and appreciation and like Naomi (male or female), you will be renewed and sustained in joy and happiness through your wisdom years.

XXXIII

The Peace and Joy of Aging

In addition to teaching the children well, which is the first investment for peace and joy in aging, you must "be true to yourself."

Be True to Yourself

As you get older, you must throw away childish things in order to wear your age gracefully. You must become honest with yourself. Stop imitating others.

Look inward to find your essence because it is imprinted into your being. The thing that keeps you alive.

It is like looking at yourself in the mirror; you will definitely recognize yourself.

My self exploratory and discovery book entitled, *Meeting and Knowing Yourself* could be useful to you, if you choose, and if you do not already have a handle on the question of who you are and your purpose on Planet Earth.

Peace comes from within you. From being contented with yourself. But you must first know that self.

XXXIV

Validate Yourself

You should no longer be looking outward to be validated.

If you are a man, do not look to other men, your boss, wife, girlfriend, money or position and power to validate you.

And if you are a woman, do not look to other women, your boss, husband, boyfriend, money or sexual control to validate you.

You cannot be validated by another person, if you do not validate yourself. And if you have already validated yourself, you will find no need to seek external validation.

You do not need another car, jet plane, new house, new wife, new husband, new girlfriend, new boyfriend to validate you.

You do not need to be a member of an exclusive club or cult to be validated You only need to acknowledge that "You Are" to be validated and to have peace within you

And if you have to put "What?" after "You Are" ("You are what?"), then you may really need to read my book, *Meeting and Knowing Yourself*, for possible assistance.

A validated person eschews inordinate power and violence against weaker and disadvantaged people because a validated self realizes that violence against others is violence against self.

Self validation is important as you get older. And once you have it, you must be true to it.

You must be true to what you call yourself. To do otherwise is to tear that self apart and place self doubt uncertainties, confusion, and chaos in the place of the calm and peace that resides therein.

The most important thing you should do as you validate yourself, if you have not already done so, is to let your Yes be Yes, and your No be No. And of course, you know that is not my quote by any imagination. The great Teacher, Philosopher and God man, Jesus Himself said it to his followers:

> "... Let your Yes be Yes, and your No, No. Anything beyond this comes from the evil one." (Matthew 5:37)

This means that anything else is being false to yourself.

Being true to yourself means you can no longer behave like a child with the excuses of your youthful years.

In his letter to the Corinthians, Paul said,

> "When I was a child, I thought like a child.
>
> I talked like a child,
>
> I reasoned like a child.
>
> When I became a man,
>
> I put childish ways behind me."
>
> (1 Corinthians 13:11)

A friend of mine proofing the manuscript of this book advised me to make it clear that Paul said "childish." not "childlike."

Childish is immature, selfish and self centered. Childlike is innocent, open, and trusting.

Paul was mindful that there is a season for everything and that aging is a season for putting away the restlessness, impetuousness, and conflict of youth for the contentment deliberateness and wisdom of the elders.

These attributes of age are what keep your soul at peace, and you should enjoy and savor them.

XXXV

Be Present for Yourself

The third attribute that gives you Peace and Joy as you get older is BEING PRESENT with yourself AT ALL TIMES.

Many adults are absent from themselves a good deal of the time.

The days go by.

The weeks go by.

The months go by.

The years go by.

And they do not know what they have done with each of these periods.

You get married.

You get divorced.

And you don't even know what happened.

Some adults scream their lungs out through the years in which they raise their kids. At that time, it looked like the period would last forever, and then one day the kids are too old to live at home. They go away to college, start a job, or get married.

Suddenly there are no children to yell at or complain about, and the adults have made no plans to be present with and live with their own selves.

Some adults in their younger years were too busy meeting deadlines, pursuing one laurel or another, that they were never present enough to enjoy the rewards of the efforts they had already put in.

How often have you held yourself back from a vacation or a trip that would have been relaxing and gratifying for you because you did not want your children, spouse, family, friends, even neighbors to complain or consider you wasteful or frivolous?

What about the article of clothing or jewelry you denied yourself because you did not have time to wear them?

"I will do this tomorrow. I will do that tomorrow."

You promised yourself repeatedly. "When I start making a little more money. When my mother-in-law leaves. When we move to a bigger house or apartment..."

Many people postpone living their own lives to its fullness. Then one day they wake up and decide that they are too old, too tired, not rich enough, or that it was not safe enough to take that vacation or wear that article of clothing.

You have one life to live, and you have not lived it. You have just existed through the time in animated absence.

This reminds me of Professor Ali Eraj, a Kenyan gynecologist of Indian descent. In his presentation to the United Nations NGO Conference on Population and Development in Bucharest in 1971, he tried to explain to the "developed" countries what life expectancy was all about for the developing nations.

"You do not understand Africa's plight," he said in a solemn voice. In the West, you live 70 years (life expectancy in the USA at that time), and then you get sick, and you die.

"In Africa we don't live at all. It takes us 30 to 40 years to die. The day we are born, we begin to die very slowly from hunger, malnutrition, infections, and all kinds of conflict. Then by 30 or 40 years, we finally get buried and they say our life expectancy is 40 years. But we never lived at all."

"How true," I thought. I never forgot the doctor's speech, and I always thought how lucky people were to live a full 70 years and then die.

But I was young then and did not really understand what living meant.

Now I believe I know better and found to my dismay that even in "Developed" countries, many people who have celebrated as many as eighty birthdays never really lived at all, either!

Too preoccupied with one fear or anxiety or the other, they journey through life absent from self.

As you age, you have an opportunity to make the changes necessary for you to be present with yourself.

XXXVI

Savor Yourself

Your very humanness is beautiful. Savor it

When you take a glass of water, don't just swallow it. Let it linger in your mouth. Feel its texture, consistency, weight, freshness. Taste it, love it and gently send it down your throat. Contemplate it as it runs down your food pipe (esophagus) into your stomach where it will join other nutrients in making you human.

Be present with your food when you eat it. Don't just chew your food, swallow and run.

Smell your food, taste your food. Think about what is on your plate, appreciate it, eat it with love, enjoy it, and marvel at how all the foods and nutrients work together to nourish you, keep you healthy and make you the beautiful person that you are.

Be present with yourself when you dress. Do not just put on your clothing because that is what is required of you.

Your clothes are the most intimate objects that you use daily. Know them and know what they do for you. Watch them go on you and transform your individual and unique naked body into whatever you wish. Enjoy them, no matter how simple, old or expensive they are.

Be present in your environment. Notice your home, where you live and sleep. Be present in the air around you. Smell the flowers and vegetation around you.

Talking about flowers...I visited one of my cousins during the Millennium Christmas and noticed there were bouquets of fresh flowers all over the house. "Who sends these flowers?" I asked him.

"ME," he said. "I pay the florist to send me whatever flower is in season weekly. You do not know it, but whenever I walk into the house, it has a different refreshing aroma. So subtle, so welcoming."

"Great idea," I said, "I am going to start doing the same for myself."

"They actually last longer than a week," he said. "Once in two weeks should be OK."

You do not have to order flowers from the florist. You can pick them yourself from your garden, or buy them from your supermarket when you do your grocery shopping.

We have already discussed in this book how important it is not only to say you love yourself, but to do loving things for yourself.

How many women there are in the real world grumbling that some husband or boyfriend has not sent them flowers, when they have not bothered to give themselves a rose petal.

And how many men scrape their pennies to impress their ladies with flowers, while they have not bothered to give themselves a gift of love and self appreciation.

Show yourself love.

Be present in your every moment, even your moments of pain. They teach you patience and wisdom and make you the sage that old age is revered for.

XXXVII

Have No Regrets

Many people go through life not paying attention to themselves, their loved ones, family, friends and colleagues; then they look back and wish they had done this and not done that.

Regrets have no positive value.

They clutter up your mind, occupying precious neuron space in your brain as you go over and over things that you cannot take back.

You can, however, remedy situations that bother you with alternate action.

Rather than preoccupying yourself with regrets, ask, "What could I have done differently?" and then, "Can I still do something about what is bothering me now?"

If the answer is Yes, do something about it and move on.

If the answer is No, forget it and move on.

The wisdom of life and creation is in moving on and not in stagnation, standing still or preservarating.

XXXVIII

Avoid Guilt

Guilt is a feeling of responsibility for wrongdoing or bad outcomes. Wrongdoing should be avoided in the first instance. If the wrongdoing occurs deliberately, you are obliged to remedy it or make restitution for it. But if you do not feel prepared to remedy the wrong, or if you are unable for any reason to provide remedy or restitution, you should not bother with the burden of guilt.

Guilt puts your body physiology in disarray, stresses your heart into hypertension and heart disease, and may fry your brain with cortisol induced by chronic stress. It may even stroke you out.

On the other hand, if the wrong doing was in error, you should bear no guilt burden although remedy and or restitution should be rendered whenever possible. This is because of the law of balance discussed earlier on.

Sometimes people feel guilty for errors or wrongdoings they have no control over. "If only I had been there he/ she might not have..."

Children, for example, sometimes feel guilty for their parents' divorce and, some carry that guilt throughout their life, when in fact there was nothing they could have done about it.

This kind of burden usually impacts them negatively at various stages in their lives. Guilt is an unnecessary burden.

It is important, therefore, for both adults and children to remedy what they can or move on. And one way to move on is to forgive all things.

XXXIX

Forgive All Things

Learning to forgive all things is one of the most important secrets of happy, healthy and wise aging.

Lack of forgiveness, like guilt, is a burden on the mind and body.

You will keep remembering that which you have not forgiven.

When some people say, "I will forgive, but I will not forget," they do not liberate themselves from the physiologic burden of remembering whatever it is they do not wish to forget.

Suppose, for example, that your best friend cheated you of some money that you had invested with him and you felt very disappointed, hurt and angry. Suppose he was sorry about his behavior, paid you the amount he borrowed and asked for forgiveness. What next?

You should forgive him completely, forget the episode and move on with your friendship.

If you said you have forgiven him but you keep reminding him of his cheating every time you have the opportunity, you will find that the feelings associated with your initial disappointment, hurt, and anger keep returning, albeit with a lesser intensity.

In addition, their stressful consequences will continue to be exhibited until you find yourself suffering from chronic stress syndrome.

You do not heal a wound when you keep pulling off the scab.

To forgive, you must forget. Forgiveness means making an offense null and void.

How Do You Learn to Forgive?

You begin with yourself.

You learn to be kind, gentle and understanding with yourself. You take time enough with yourself to know what you really like, what makes you happy, what makes you sad, and you learn to understand why you do what you do and then learn to forgive yourself.

Most likely, when you forgive yourself of a wrongdoing or an error, you do not go about reminding yourself about your previous mistakes.

Forgiving yourself is important because, as with love, you cannot give what you do not have. You cannot forgive others when you do not forgive yourself.

Forgiving yourself liberates you to forgive others.

The Biblical advice to "...first take the plank out of your eye, and then you will see more clearly to remove the speck from your brother's eye" (Luke 6:42), is not only about judging others; it is also about how to forgive others.

Guilt results when you have not forgiven yourself of whatever you feel guilty about. And as we discussed above, guilt is negative energy that ultimately destroys your physiology. It should be avoided. This is why you must forgive yourself.

Once you learn to forgive yourself, it is easier to forgive others.

Forgiveness is so important that it is the only grace of God that is conditional on your behavior.

"Forgive us our trespasses

As we forgive those who trespass against us..." (The Lord's Prayer, Matthew 6:12)

This is because forgiveness is the liberator of the mind, body, and spirit which puts us in the mode to receive all the other graces like love, faith, and hope. It is in this mode that we are able to live life in its fullness.

There is wisdom in forgiving all things. Practice forgiveness and teach the youth the same.

XL

Life Begins at 40

Earlier in this book, I promised you that I will be discussing what we mean by the adage, "Life begins at 40."

This is a good time to do so.

We know that we have been alive from birth until the present, so it must not be the physical life as we know it, that we are referring to when we say life begins at forty.

Which life, then, is it that begins at forty?

We find when we compare life experiences, that in general, there is a definite personal crisis around age 40, give or take three years, for everyone who lives long enough. This seems to be a universal human life experience without regard for race, color, culture, religion, geographic location or level of education.

It is also observed, that within the seven years of 37, 38, 39, 40, 41, 42, and 43, expected or not, desired or not, most people have a major change in their life that affects the status or direction of their life, as they knew it up to that time.

XLI

Once Upon a Woman's Change of Life

Once upon a time, people called this startling change, "Middle Age Crisis."

They explained it away for women: that the children had grown up and flown the coop. They claimed that since the main function of women was sexual, they had been used up, and had nothing more to offer.

As for unmarried women, they were so frustrated with their manless life that they were no use anyway.

And those poor women who were married but had no children, well, they were being punished for some offense that they had not admitted to, like being unfaithful to their husbands.

In their perception, at that time, with nothing more to do, it was an appropriate time for women to suffer depression, feel useless, and get abandoned or at least benignly neglected by their husbands of several years.

Soon it would be time for them to begin to shrivel, become witches, fall down, break a hip, and get thrown into a nursing home where they would shrill and shrink, become eccentric, ultimately lose control of their body functions and die.

Later on, science came along to explain that the changes, especially those of sexual desirability, were due to hormonal changes, especially the estrogen drop that accompanied the so-called "change of life."

They called it "menopause," and then tried to explain or blame everything else that happened after that on the loss of these and other hormones.

Science was willing to help women become more "functional" by replacing their waning hormones. This would help them continue to provide their usual sexual services to their men.

Science or tradition, the function of the woman was the same: "Provide sexual services to your man, or else..."

XLII

Once Upon a Man's Change of Life

For men, age 40 traditionally heralded the beginning of the loss of virility and sexual potency.

It was believed that sexual potency made a man a man, and since he did not want to give up his sexual image after his wife has become conspicuously sexually undesirable, he sought younger women to awaken his weakened libido.

Sometimes, he flirted with his secretary, a student or just the neighborhood kids. Occasionally, he had an affair serious enough to send his wife packing.

He, too, was fighting his physical profile—bulging abdomen, hairs growing in his ears and gray hair cropping on his sexy chest. How insulting.

He was usually the breadwinner and the one who made the rules, so though his libido might have declined a bit, he was not useless. Unlike the woman, in fact, he was very much needed because he was the father and head of family.

Later on, scientists in their growing knowledge discovered that the man's decrease in virility was due to the male hormone testosterone, decreasing as he came around the 40-year bend.

He too, had what they called middle age crisis. The scientists could help him so that he would continue to be sexually active. They would give him testosterone replacement therapy. (That was before the days of Viagra.)

Everything was about sexual satisfaction.

Change of life and its impact on sexual activities by adults at the time were perceived, especially by men with the big male ego, as a deprivation of what was rightfully his.

Before the days of Viagra, while his wife struggled with rejection and rapid psychological decline, the man looked for a younger woman to marry to prop himself up for a few more years.

He did not go to the nursing home quite so quickly. In fact, he had a good chance of being buried by the younger wife after a heart attack or stroke as a result of pushing the sex and power stuff a little too hard.

By his sudden death time, it was not unusual for the younger wife to have produced a few little kids of her own, to inherit his money or property so that the cycle can continue.

That was supposed to be the normal pattern: Midlife Crisis and then downhill.

The purpose of life was for sex and reproduction, everybody was taught, and once those functions had been fulfilled and sexual dissatisfaction was imposed on the male by partial or complete impotence, there was no point "hanging around" life.

Evidence seemed to say this, traditions said so, too, and scientists provided explanations for those perceptions.

But those perceptions and explanations were wrong. Very wrong.

LXIII

There is No Middle Age Crisis

No middle age crisis exists that spirals downward.

There is a new beginning, a birthing into the spiritual phase of life that begins at about age 40, give or take three years.

The first phase of physical life as we know it on planet Earth, is about physical development and maturity in preparation for the second phase, which is the spiritual phase; which is a preparation for the third and universal phase of being.

Recall that before the physical phase, most of us were nine months in our mothers' wombs in preparation for our earthly birthing. But the egg that formed us with the help of our father's sperm had been in our mothers' ovaries from their own births, and before then in their mothers all the way back to the first woman to birth a child.

This is not the book to discuss where the first mother and father came from.

However, we shall take a close look at this birthing process into the second stage of our fives.

Sex is a Carrot

If our life was simply about reproduction and survival of the species, we should be like most animals, programmed by instinct to mate in heat only.

Or if sex was so extremely compelling to us, we should act like dogs and have no rules about committing to one partner or feeling jealous if our partner mates with other people.

We are not quite one or the other. We are a thinking and reasoning species, with free will to make choices.

And because we tend to commit better when there is incentive, we were designed with the carrot of pleasurable sex to increase our incentive to reproduce.

Most women would not design reproduction of the species the way it currently is if they had been consulted about it.

And a lot of men would not be bothered with fathering children, either, if there were no pleasures in the act of insemination.

Sex is the carrot provided to lure both men and women into the act that would propagate humanity, while placing them on the starting line of life's journey toward spirituality and universality.

However, this sexual incentive is designed to terminate at the birthing into spirituality, when we are supposed to shift our focus from the outward and physical to the inward and spiritual

The mundane to the sublime,

The intangible to the tangible.

But the carrot was so sweet, especially for the male who knew nothing else to that point that he was reluctant to give it up. And rightly so.

Why would any one wish to give up such a pleasant act, especially since the burden of bearing the product of the act is the woman's?

No, he would not give it up without a fight!

But the Great Designer, who knows that life's journey has a greater mission than its physical pleasures, anticipated this reluctance to give up the carrot and instituted the gradual withdrawal of these incentives, by putting pauses on the road, as we have previously discussed in this book.

In addition to the placing of hormonal and physical pauses, something radical had to change to draw our attention away from the physical to Phase Two.

A baby in the womb might become so comfortable with the life and environment known to that point that he might not wish to enter our physical world for Phase One of life's journey. But he does not have the option to remain in the womb indefinitely. He has to be birthed by force, whether he likes it or not, whether he believes in the world he is getting into or not.

If he is not birthed when the time is due there are serious consequences for him and his mother.

Similarly, an adult at age 40, give or take three years, has to be birthed into the spiritual phase by force, whether he or she likes it or not, and whether he or she believes in it or not.

If he or she is not birthed, like the baby, there are serious consequences for him or her.

XLIV

Birthing into a New Beginning at 40

Just as the newborn baby enters the physical phase of life kicking and screaming even though he is not really aware of what he is doing, many adults enter the spiritual phase of their life kicking and screaming although they, too, are not really aware of what they are doing.

Looking back now I realize that I, too, entered my birthing at 40 screaming and resisting.

For the amount of fun I was having in the physical Phase One of my life, no one was going to drag me into the spiritual phase of life without a fight. But when you got to go, you got to go.

I will tell you my own age 40 story later. For now, let's share the story of BJ's birthing at 40.

Status Quo is Good; Don't Rock the Boat

I suppose that for every example of the birthing experience of men and women at age 40 that I give, you probably have several dozen examples you could supply.

In any case, BJ was a tall, handsome, and fine gentleman with enviable attributes.

BJ was real.

He was 45 years old and had been married since age 22 to the same woman. They had a son and three daughters, aged seven to eighteen years.

BJ worked as a builder while his wife was a full-time homemaker. On his fortieth birthday he took his wife out for a celebration dinner. When they came back home, the wife suggested that since they could not have any more infants, she would not mind working to make additional income for the family. BJ thought that was a good idea.

Soon the wife was working in a shopping mall.

Labor Pains Come Slowly at First

Three months later, BJ noticed that his wife was returning home late. He monitored her and soon found her kissing another man in his car in the parking lot of the mall.

BJ was shattered. How could she do a thing like that? When he confronted her with his observation she got angry and asked for a divorce.

A confused BJ did not know what to do. He had been faithful to his own marriage vows. He adored his wife and their children. He could not imagine a life without her. But before he could figure out a reconciliation program including marriage counseling, the wife moved out of the house, leaving him behind with the four children.

BJ, now a single father of four at 40, plunged into depression. He felt abandoned, betrayed, lonely, and ashamed.

He had no extended family to talk to, and he could not turn to his church community because the man his wife was dating was a member of his church congregation.

He now had to juggle his construction work with cooking and cleaning, making sure his underage children went to school on time, and that he was around to receive them after school. He also had to appear in court for divorce proceedings.

He felt less than a man every time he went to court and found his wife with the other man. "What did that man have to offer his wife that he did not have?" he wondered.

His wife was a goddess of beauty, as far as he was concerned. "How could such a goddess fall into the hands of an evil man?" he asked himself.

It was unbearable. "I never laid a hand on her in our twenty years of marriage," he sobbed. Life would not have been worth living if not because of the great love he had for his children. But the stress of everything was getting the better of him.

Soon his job started to suffer. His construction business started to decline. He had several houses on rent for extra income, but he was too depressed, tired or disinterested to maintain them. He started to put them on sale, one at a time. Before he knew it, four years had passed, and he had sold his business and had no money to feed four children and himself.

While all this was happening, he kept hoping his wife would change her mind and call everything a mistake so they could start afresh, but that never happened.

Birthing Pain Ends Just when it is Getting Too Much to Bear

By his 44th birthday, embittered BJ had become so antisocial and so distrustful that the whole world had become enemy territory for him. No friends, no one to trust. He was always on guard.

Then one day, after getting one bill too many, he decided he had had enough. He called an old friend. “I have had it,” he said. “I am going to send my children to their mother, sell my house and go to another state to start again. I do not understand why I am suffering, and my ex-wife is enjoying herself. I am the one who is abandoned, and I am the one paying the price. I can’t take it any more.”

The last sentence, “I can’t take it any more,” scared the friend because she thought BJ might be contemplating suicide.

“Please see me, BJ,” the friend requested.

After the two old friends had a long session together, the friend asked BJ, “Have you learned the lesson that your wife leaving you was supposed to teach you?”

“I am not sure if I have learned anything. All I know is that I have suffered too long for what is not my fault and I am tired of this pain. I want it to stop.”

“The time has come for the pain to stop,” the friend replied. “If you would, take your attention away from your ex-wife and focus it on yourself. The pain is inside you, not outside you. Look inside you to find what you need to heal yourself. It is not that someone abandoned you that is still hurting you. It is that you abandoned yourself.

“You placed so much importance on what your wife was providing for you and what she represented for your social status that you are trying to define yourself from outside yourself.

“But you cannot define yourself from outside yourself, because you reside inside yourself, not outside.

"To heal, you should begin by forgiving your ex-wife, her lover, and everyone else. And above all, forgive yourself for being absent from yourself."

Pain of Birthing Stops when the Shift is Made

Several months later his friend invited him to attend a retreat. At the retreat the friend asked him how he was coping with his life.

> "I have returned to myself," he said. "I am so much happier now. Once I decided to forgive my wife—my ex-wife, I mean—and the whole gang of cheats, it felt like a big weight had been lifted from my shoulders. Then I started spending thirty minutes by myself each day in silence, doing nothing.
>
> "It is amazing how these 'do nothing times' quieted me and made me calm and serene. I do not know how it happened, but I suddenly realized that I was talking to someone inside me during these quiet moments. We were holding conversations on just about anything that interested me.
>
> "Then it clicked This was my spirit! It had been wanting to capture my attention for so long, but I was too hung up on my wife to pay attention.
>
> "I don't know how I could have missed it for so long and gone through all that pain if the answer was so simple.
>
> "Now I do not do anything without discussing it with my spirit. I have started rebuilding my business and am no longer under any serious debt pressures.

"Yes, I have started dating again, but I am exercising self restraint.

"My ex-wife still works in the mall, and from time to time I pass by there and say hello to her. She is still the mother of our lovely children, and I still love her but have no more pain."

"And what do you see in your future?" the friend asked.

"Beginning my passion, which is sculpting. Who knows, some day I may have an exhibition!"

Spiritual Birthing Propels its Own Change

I tell the story of BJ to make the point that the so called "Middle Age Crisis," which is actually a birthing into the spiritual phase of life at 40, does not announce itself as such, but invariably propels the individual into shifting attention from the outside and physical self, to the inside and spiritual self.

BJ's birthing took almost five years, but he has now begun the second phase of his journey, like many did before him, feeling contented and mellow. At 45 years, he is just beginning to understand his mission.

XLV

Premature Death

This second story is about Jessica, who at age 41, lost her 42-year-old husband in a car crash.

Jessica and her husband Nat had the perfect life and marriage. He was a professor and she was an administrator in the same university. Together, they made a handsome amount of money for themselves and their two sons and two daughters.

They were still so much in love after 17 years of marriage that they still cooked and cleaned up after meals together, laughing and kidding their way through everything.

Then one foggy day, while driving home from an official assignment, Nat ran his Volvo car into a parked truck and died on the spot. Horror.

"I only kissed him before he left. I did not know that that was the final kiss. I have lost my best friend," Jessica sobbed.

After Nat's funeral, Jessica went into deep depression.

She started wearing black or dark clothes, stopped socializing and participating in university community activities and taking care of her beautiful self.

She worried about everything, especially about her children, job, and finances.

To complicate issues, some of Nat's friends tried to seduce her while she was still mourning her husband's death, and that made her afraid.

She did not want to continue to live in their house without Nat. It held too much memory for her. Besides, she could no longer afford the mortgage. She felt the university had become a hostile environment and changed jobs. She took a job in another university, in a different geographic location, far away from her pains.

Run as she could, she could not escape her heartache, which was worse at right, when she was lying alone in bed

Sleep eluded her night after night. Then her blood pressure started to rise until she needed to see the doctor for hypertension medication.

She started to see herself as a widow suffering insomnia and hypertension with four children to raise alone. Her future was shut, as far as she was concerned.

One night, about a year and half after Nat's death, while lying awake sobbing as usual, her telephone rang. It was an old friend from college. She never really liked him while they were in college and when he dropped out of college, she completely forgot about him. From his perspective, in or out of college, Mark had always fancied Jessica.

Excited to hear from an old friend, Jessica enthusiastically acknowledged Mark.

"Sorry to hear you lost Nat," Mark said.

That was all Jessica needed to start pouring her heart out to Mark about the loss of her husband.

"I have always wanted to marry you," Mark's voice broke through Jessica's stories. "I have called to tell you that I do not want to lose this chance again. Jessica, would you marry me?"

Silence in the air waves.

"Jessica, did you hear me?"

"What in the world are you talking about?" Jessica queried as she stared wide eyed into the telephone.

"Jessica, would you marry me? Yes or No? That's all I want to know."

"Yes," Jessica replied.

Silence.

"Did I hear you say Yes, Jessica?" a surprised Mark screamed in disbelief.

"Yes, I will marry you," Jessica replied calmly and then put down the telephone receiver.

The next morning as Jessica was getting her children ready for school, Mark was ringing the doorbell. He had driven three hundred miles overnight to claim his new bride!

Jessica, who thought that the past night's discussion was a dream, could not believe her eyes. After polite exchanges, she asked Mark to come into the house.

Once inside the house, with the children off to school, Mark went on his knees. "Jessica, I have always wanted to many you. I know that you have forgotten all about me, but I have followed your progress from a distance since your marriage twenty years ago. I have four children of my own from my failed marriage. If you do not mind them, I want you to be my wife."

As if in a trance, Jessica said, "Yes, I will marry you." They both stared at each other in disbelief.

Marriage arrangements were made at frightening speed. Two weeks after their meeting, Mark and Jessica were husband and wife.

Mark continued to live and work three hundred miles away. He said he did not want Jessica to relocate or change her job after her recent move. He called her every day and visited her almost every weekend.

Mark was happy with his fulfilled ambition. Jessica was mad at herself.

She was married but still alone at night. She cried because of Nat. She cried because of her children. She cried because she was ashamed of her senseless decision to marry a man she did not even know.

"I don't know what came over me. I do not know who married Mark, but it is not me. I can't stand the man touching me. I dread the weekends these days and dread Mark's coming because he bulldozes over everything. I feel so dirty." Jessica confided to a girlfriend, as she sobbed quietly after one of Mark's weekend visits. I wish I had died with Nat."

Mark's agenda did not include Nat's memory, so he promptly removed all of Nat's photographs from display in Jessica's house and replaced them with his, or their wedding photographs. Jessica did not like the arrangement, but she felt helpless.

She had lost control of her life. More than that, she had lost her very self.

Jessica continued to spiral downward for two years. She thought less and less of herself and barely hung onto life because of her children.

Suicidal thoughts became a daily obsession.

One day while planning what she would write in her suicide note for her children, a thought entered her mind "Who are you running away from? How would you explain all this to Nat if you died and met him again?"

The thought made her realize that she could not run away from herself. If she died she would still die with herself.

What happens after she dies? Would she still be hurting? Would she be happier after dying? Would she still exist after dying? If she disappeared completely and had no conscious existence anywhere, what were all the physical and emotional experiences for anyway?

The more she pondered these questions, the calmer she became and the less she thought about suicide.

After that experience, she found herself pondering the meaning of her life and the purpose for which she had lived.

Very gradually, she began to feel a need to explore the holy books for answers. She was an avid reader. She read the Christian Bible, the Muslim Khoran, and Confucious's Analects.

Where did her sadness come from? Her children were doing well. They were well behaved and studied hard at school. They were exemplary.

She had a good job and was well compensated for her work.

Mark was not Nat, but he was her husband and except for his sexual demands, he allowed her all the freedom she wished.

So, why was she sad? Why was she still hurting? And who was hurting her?

The shocking answer came: "Me." Jessica is the one hurting Jessica. Jessica was entirely externally focused.

She thought that the joy and happiness she had experienced with Nat was given to her by Nat and that when Nat died, he took the joy and happiness with him.

Though her marriage to Mark was an irrational decision, Mark was not a total disaster and did not require a divorce for remedy. He had not relieved her misery, but he was not the cause of it. She, Jessica, was the cause of Jessica's misery. How?

She had lost her sense of self. Jessica did not really know who Jessica was. Was she the widowed mother of four? One of them was now in college and doing well. Was she Mark's wife? She certainly did not feel like a wife, not like she did with Nat. Was she a university administrator? She had been that for years. Nothing new.

Had she exhausted herself? Completed all she was born to do in life? Who was Jessica anyway?

She had not been a religious person and professed no particular faith, but each day as she confronted herself with the question; "Who was Jessica anyway?" she found herself spending more and more time listening to her inner dialog. And the more she held these dialogs, the less sad she felt

She started to smile again.

A radiance returned to her face with a fullness of peace. Mark thought it was magic!

"About time the sun came out," Mark told her in one of his weekend visits. "We have been married for two years now. For a while, I thought you had forgotten how to be alive."

"No, I did not forget how to be alive. I just did not know which part of me was supposed to be alive. Now I know and everything else is all right," Jessica said as her voice rang out in laughter.

That was the story of Jessica's birthing at forty. Now, I will share what happened to me at forty.

XLVI

Becoming

My life at forty started at age 39.

In my early thirties I had a fibroid tumor that was being watched by my doctor.

Then, suddenly it started to grow like a coconut fruit so that by age 39, it was so large that it started to cause me severe lower abdominal pain.

The tumor had to go.

The surgery was simple enough. However, on the fifth day after my surgery, just before discharge, I found my bed sheet wet. I could not figure out where the water came from.

I called the nurse's attention to my wet sheets and after examining them, she said she would tell the doctor during his morning rounds.

Being a doctor myself, I feared the worst, but would not dare think of it.

The dreaded news came after my doctor examined me. Something was wrong with my bladder. I had to go back to surgery for repairs.

On hearing that proposition, an unbelievable fear physically took over my whole body from my hair down to my toenails.

I had thick tears hanging on my eyes that wouldn't even drop. I had two young children at home. I was sure that if I went back to surgery, I would die. Yet the thought of leaving the hospital without bladder control was unthinkable to me.

Very slowly I said to my doctor, "I did not tell my children I was going to die. If I had bid them good-bye I would not have minded dying. I just cannot die like that, I will have to go back home to tell my children I am going to die, and then I will come back for the operation and death."

My doctor, who knew me very well and who had been one of my teachers during my internship year, said "OK."

I went back home and was incapacitated for about nine months. I had apparently had some nerve injury during the spinal anesthesia for the fibroid operation. It had affected my bladder and both sides of my thighs, so that one was numb and the other so sensitive that the touch of my clothes almost felt like pain.

Since it was a nerve injury, surgery in those days could not have helped me. It's a good thing I did not consent to surgery.

While at home, like all indisposed people, I prayed, I changed my diet, and I waited for a miracle.

Before the fibroid operation, which was the third surgery of my life, I was a restless go getter, involved in everything—tennis, squash, jogging, dancing, traveling, and whatever else a beautiful and healthy young woman in her thirties would enjoy doing.

Then at age thirty-nine, I was forced to pause and take a good look at everything in life.

In the subsequent nine months while my nerve injury healed and I recovered my bladder control and my thighs started to feel normal again, I had slowed down enough to actually begin to hear the quiet sound of my spirit. But I was not truly paying attention.

I was so enthusiastic when my 40th birthday armed that I celebrated it in two continents, partying from Europe to Africa.

I continued to charge on with my physical focused youthful exuberance until age 42, when, after a particularly good vacation in the Los Angeles area, I got on a flight from Los Angeles via New York City to London.

Everything was going well for me.

I was flying first class, drinking champagne and all that came with it, when suddenly the taste in my mouth changed.

It was about 2 a.m. We were flying over the Atlantic Ocean en route to London. As the taste in my mouth changed, I heard a voice in my ears say, "Your spirit does not like alcohol."

When I first heard it, I thought it was a figment of my imagination.

I ignored the voice and asked the stewardess to give me more champagne. She did. I took a sip of my new drink. It tasted like sawdust.

I was wondering what to do with the drink, when I heard again, "Your spirit does not like alcohol."

Irritated by whatever was talking to me or putting the idea in my head, I said more or less to myself, "How come? Where has my spirit been all the time I was enjoying the best of California and French wines I could get my hands on in Los Angeles?"

I was not drunk. I had been drunk only once in my life and that was the summer after my junior year in college. Here's what happened.

After completing our summer program, a group of us went partying in a tour boat on the Mississippi Missouri Rivers, with gallons of Yago wine for good measure.

No, I was not drunk. And I was not going to let any spirit threaten my little pleasures, I thought.

I called on the stewardess once more and requested that she remove my champagne glass and get me some dry white wine in its place.

Once again she politely replaced my drink. Just as I was about to take a sip of this drink, I heard in the loudest voice, "Your spirit does not like alcohol."

This time I was so piqued by the interruptions of my quiet that I shouted back, "Yes, I hear. My spirit does not like alcohol."

Why would my spirit say it did not like alcohol?

Did it have to deny me of the one thing I considered real classy in my *novo riche* repertoire?

Why did it not ask me to give up something I did not like? Smoking for example.

I needed to meet this "spirit" that does not like alcohol. Mediation was the direct route for deliberate meeting with my Spirit. I went for it, thanks to Peter's book.

To my amazement the first thing I found was that my Spirit, like Jesus, is real. That my Spirit is the presence of God in me which keeps me alive, protects me and guides me. It tells me the right thing to do, but sometimes my mind and brain overrule its advice, to my avoidable distress.

Next, I found that my Spirit is as stubborn in getting me to do the right thing as I am stubborn in wanting to do the contrary.

Finally, I found that if I listened to my Spirit I always made the right choices and stayed in a state of joy.

My Ego initially liked to confront my Spirit, but invariably I ended up in physical, mental and emotional pain. Then I found that complete submission of my Ego to the Spirit of God in me was the answer for pain relief in me.

With the submission of my Ego to my Spirit I began the spiritual phase of my life's journey. And Oh, what a journey!

Now I understand, that knowing God and becoming Christlike in submission, is life's mission, for me at least and that my job of doctoring is actually part of this becoming of the healing grace of Christ.

Could I extend this understanding to others? Is it possible that each of us is here to express in our own field and life, if we choose, an aspect of Christ's image? Like the farmer is expressing Christ the feeder of multitudes?

I do not know the answer, but I know that since my Spirit and not my Ego started guiding me I live in the presence of God. And where God lives is called Heaven.

XLVII

A Journey of Faith

Faith is confidence in the unknown. Belief in events and conditions yet to occur in the future. Trust in a person, place or thing that has no material evidence.

Faith is not about belief or lack of belief in God It is about us and the way we live.

The whole of life is an act of faith. Life as we know it on this planet Earth is impossible without faith.

In your latent state in your mother's womb, though not consciously aware of it, you must have had faith (belief, confidence, trust) in your mother, that she would carry you through the pregnancy into a viable baby and human being.

Those whose mothers broke the faith of their conception were aborted and are not here to read these words.

After birth you had faith in your parents or their substitute to feed you when you were hungry, clothe you to keep you warm, change you when you were wet or soiled, and comfort you when you had noxious stimulation.

Though you did know it as a baby, you submitted completely to your parents because you needed them for your physical survival and comfort.

If they broke the faith, you would become an abandoned, neglected or abused child.

You Need Faith to Go to School

When you started elementary school, you were still mostly ignorant and unaware of the reality around you, but somehow, you and your parents or guardians believed the teachers in your school would teach you and make you knowledgeable.

You might not have liked some of the things that happened to you in school, but you had faith that the education was for your ultimate good. It would help you get into high school and maybe go beyond.

If your school authorities or teachers broke the faith, your education might be truncated and you could be traumatized for life.

You needed faith to get into high school and college.

When you enrolled in high school or college, you did not know if you would graduate. You did not even know if you would die first, but you believed you would graduate and move on; hence the effort on your part to go through the rigors of education.

You also Need Faith to be a Farmer

Suppose you did not wish to pursue education and became a farmer instead.

When you plant your grain or whatever, you do not know if you will have a harvest, but you believe you will. You have faith that the soil, the weather, and the interplay of pests, other elements and your labor will produce a harvest for you, but you do not know it. Every moment of your life is an act of faith.

When you get up each morning to go to school or work, the school and work places are your future for that day. You do not know If you will arrive at your destination, but you have the faith you will, and you usually do.

There is no end to examples of how you express your faith every moment of your life.

If you get on a plane to fly from one place to the other, you express so much faith it is impossible to list all of your points of faith here. For example, you believe in the pilot, whom you may or may not know, that he would fly the plane safely to your destination. You believe in the physical plane itself, that is a sound vehicle to take you to your destination. You believe in the engineers who designed and built the plane, that they put everything in its proper place and position. You believe in the principles of aerodynamics, whether you understand them or not, that they would operate as stated to make the plane take off, fly, and land safely and so on.

Without faith you would be filled with anxiety and paralyzed from all actions and die.

XLVIII

Anxiety is Born When Faith is Absent

If you got on a plane and had no faith (confidence, belief, trust) that you would get to your destination, you would become anxious.

If you left your house in the morning for school or work and had no faith you would arrive at your destination, you would become anxious.

If you planted your seeds or seedlings in the farm and had no faith there would be harvest, you would become anxious.

Anxiety results when there is doubt about an anticipated outcome.

We are born with absolute faith

And educated into anxiety.

If you went to bed at night, and had no faith that you would wake up the next morning, you would be so anxious, you would not be able to steep; unless it is from exhaustion.

Watch a little baby or child sleep.

Faith is what you see as the innocence in his face. He has absolute faith in his environment and care givers.

He sleeps with abandon.

Introduce a tale of terror or a horror movie or a fight before the child goes to sleep and he gets a nightmare.

Innocent is lost

While

Wisdom is out of reach

The epidemic of social anxiety syndrome that is said to have overtaken the people at the dawn of the new millennium is evidence of the absence of faith (confidence, belief, trust) in everything in society.

It cannot be resolved by pills, despite the commercial advertisements.

XLIX

We Are Educated into Anxiety

The child is a model of the faith you need while still ignorant, and the adult at forty and thereafter should be a model of faith in the presence of knowledge.

As you get older, if you combine knowledge with faith, you will go towards wisdom.

Unfortunately, our educational systems and methods are designed to remove faith from us, and replace it with what some people call a healthy dose of skepticism. Scientific proof. Materialization.

The irony is that once there is proof or materialization, there is no need for the type of faith you had as a child. While our educational systems appear appropriate for our physical and material world, it helps to fixate us on the physical and material states.

We begin to need the evidence for proof. We need a large bank account for proof we have money. We turn to big houses, cars, boats and jet planes for proof of material wealth. Large reserves of grain in the barn are proof of our farm harvest.

Material evidence and proofs confirm our evidence-based knowledge and make the need for faith unnecessary.

The result of this is that may people grow up with lots of physical knowledge and no faith in the unseen, the unmaterialized or the future, even though our scientists tell us that over ninety percent of our universe is unmaterialized Dark Matter.

And when they are unable to demonstrate or materialize the future to prove its existence, they get anxious. They develop doubt and begin to speculate instead of believing because they have been educated out of faith.

When a critical mass of people become anxious because of their doubts and uncertainties, it becomes a social norm.

This norm of coercive anxiety is then paraded by talk show television programs and the so called pundits on a daily basis as signs of a dysfunctional society.

This puts us further away from our beginning child- like faith and confidence.

L

We Demand Evidence-Based Knowledge

At birth, though we have no recollection of our existence before birth, we can formulate our future fairly easily because the evidence is all around us. We see our parents or guardians and materially successful people around us. We can model ourselves after any of them.

This seems realistic.

So we plan to become like our parents. We set the goals to get there and we work toward the goals.

By age forty, give or take three years, when we get a rebirth into the second phase of life, we have been so educated into evidence based knowledge and materialization that the spiritual phase of life appears unrealistic and no longer makes "scientific sense."

We have been educated out of faith. We are no longer children, and have since forgotten how to trust, believe or have confidence in the unseen that is yet to come.

We look around for the physical and concrete evidence of those who had crossed the forty year bend before us, and we see them deteriorating physically. Voila! That is the proof!

"If you age, after forty you will break your hip and die."

We do not want to break our hips, and we do not really want to die, so we proceed into the subsequent years with depression and sadness and little or no expectations.

We make no plans because we know we would die sooner or later. Probably sooner, because each day we live brings us closer to our dying day.

We live as we wait to die rather than as we wait to achieve.

We start grappling for straws to hold onto, for—

As the newborn knows not from whence he came

The adult at forty knows not where he goeth

We live as if dying were the purpose of life, an end in itself.

Our priest, pastor, rabbi, imam, or other religious leader tells us about life after death. They tell us we will not die. (But the physical evidence tells us differently.) They tell us we need faith to take us to the life after death.

We are baffled, even angry, that they are telling us to "regress" to our childhood faith, to begin to trust again like helpless infants. That cannot be right. The evidence is there. Children have no power. When we become like children again, we would lose the power that took us so long to acquire.

No, we conclude, this faith thing is for the weak, poor, hungry, and powerless.

We stumble through phase two of our life with no clear vision of our future and no definite plans.

Then our friends begin to die one by one. One gets cancer and dies; the other suffers a heart attack and yet another gets Alzheimer's and becomes a zombie.

We become anxious and afraid. Remember anxiety and fear can only be born in the absence of faith. We have no faith, because we have been educated out of it.

What are we going to do?

(You may wish to re-read the first chapters in this book, "Conquering Your Fears," and "Where Do You Get Your Fears?")

LI

Faith Added to Knowledge Creates Wisdom

Life is a process. It has no beginning and no end. It is always becoming.

The human experience is part of life. This means that we are all individually and collectively in the process of becoming.

We are traveling toward the universality phase, but we never quite arrive there. To arrive means to stop the traveling, the becoming. This is not possible, because that will change the very essence of life.

It is this constant becoming that the scientists call evolution. However, it does not mean that an amoeba becomes an antelope or that Dolly the sheep becomes a leopard (This could be the thesis for another book.)

For now, we note that there is order in the Universe of creation but not from the big bang of anything. In our evidence based knowledge, a big bang of anything never produced any order, just deformation of sequence. Even then, the big bang theory is an act of faith. No human or animal saw or heard the big bang. And those who propose it as the cause of our universe and life, do so in trust and belief (faith).

We live on an earth that is constantly rotating on its axis and revolving around the sun. On it, seasons come and go and come again, but no season ever repeats itself in the same exact way. There is progression. The earth, like us, is also becoming.

LII

Knowledge, Wisdom, and Faith

Wisdom comes in our understanding of the process of our becoming, and in applying that knowledge to solving problems that confront us, our society, country or world in the present or future.

Wisdom is the sound application of knowledge in faith to the conduct of our affairs.

For our purposes, we shall define knowledge as the understanding we gained by actual experience. The dictionary says that "knowledge could be empirical, material and/or that derived by inference or interpretation."

The same Webster's dictionary also defines wisdom, as "sound judgment and ability to apply what has been acquired mentally (knowledge) to the conduct of one's affairs."

It takes time to acquire knowledge, formally or informally. This is why you need age for wisdom.

King Solomon the Wise

King Solomon, merely a boy when he became king of Israel, was aware that he did not have the age advantage on his side to have accumulated enough wisdom to make sound judgments for his subjects, so he requested God in his dream, to grant him wisdom.

With wisdom granted him, King Solomon was able to make the classic judgment that is repeated by all people interested in wisdom and justice.

According to the story, two women who lived in the same room delivered their infant sons three days apart.

The first woman, who had the older baby, claimed that while they slept at night, the second woman inadvertently lay on top of her new infant, and he died from suffocation. The second woman, then took the dead infant and exchanged it with the first woman's living child while both mother and child were in deep sleep.

When the first woman woke up she found the dead infant by her side, next to her breast. She was naturally distraught. But at daybreak and on closer examination, she discovered the dead baby was not hers. She wanted her living baby back from the second woman, but the second woman would not return the live baby, claiming the living baby was hers.

When the case was presented to the Wisdom King Solomon, he asked his aides to get a sword and split the living child into two equal parts and give one half to each woman. They would probably do the same with the dead infant.

But the first woman, filled with compassion and love for the living chid, cried and begged the king, "Please, my lord, give her (the second woman) the living baby! Don't kill him!"

But the other woman said, "Neither I nor you shall have him. Cut him in two!"

Then the king gave his ruling: "Give the living baby to the first woman. Do not kill him. She is the mother." (1 Kings 3:26-27)

King Solomon's sound judgment was based on knowledge of human behavior and faith (belief, confidence) that this behavior would be reproducible under the right circumstances.

The king did not know for sure what the mother of the dead baby would say or do, but he had confidence (faith) that the nature of human behavior would reveal itself when the time and circumstances were right.

The Stock Market and Faith

The stock market is another example of the interplay of wisdom, faith, and knowledge.

By studying stock market trends, based on the actual experience (knowledge) of what has happened in the past months and years, the stock broker invests in the present or future stocks, with the belief and confidence (faith) that the stock market trends are reproducible.

This sound judgment (wise decision) usually results in financial gains for him and his clients.

Like Solomon, the stockbroker does not know for sure what the stock market will do; he bases his decision or advice to others in his faith that the future will bring the same results that knowledge from actual experience in the past has shown or demonstrated.

The Weather Forecaster and Faith

The weather forecaster is yet another example of a person whose profession is an act of faith. (I won't use the medical profession as my third example, because everyone knows that medicine is the epitome of professional acts of faith.) Yes, let us talk about the weather forecaster.

When the weather forecaster looks at the satellite images of hot or cold fronts, moist or dry currents etc., and predicts a winter storm, a hurricane, typhoon or whatever, for the next hours, days, weeks or even years; he is not in the future. His faith is.

Like King Solomon and the stock broker, the weather forecaster does not know for sure what will happen in a few hours, days, weeks or years. But he believes (faith), based on the cumulated data (knowledge), that the weather, at an expected future date and time, will behave in a certain way.

In summary, what we call evidence-based knowledge or scientific proof is actually the materialization (in the present) of what was faith (the future of the past).

We need faith to be wise.

The educational system that strips us of faith, in the name of evidence based or scientific proof, deprives us of wisdom and opens us up to the ridicule of folly.

It follows, therefore, that if by our wisdom years we fail to soundly apply our cumulated knowledge in handling our own affairs, we open ourselves to the ridicule of the folly implied in the adage, “A fool at forty is a fool forever.”

When society accumulates a critical mass of follies (bad judgment among the elders, they, the elders, lose the respect of the youth because they become like fools to the youth.

LIII

Faith Requires a Photograph of the Future

One of my favorite television evangelists, Dr. Mike Murdock, says that "Faith requires a picture or photograph for fulfillment." By this he means, as we wrote earlier in this book, that you need a vision of your goal before you can achieve it.

Because so many of us get stuck in the physical stage of our life, phase one, we are unable not only to enjoy, but even to see through the spiritual stage, phase two, into the infinite future to the universal stage of our life or consciousness.

Many perseverate on the physical infirmities that come with advancing age and miss the spiritual growth that transforms us into the glory of the universality state.

We need a picture of that glorious future to focus on.

How do we get it?

The Great Historic Figure, Jesus Christ, the Divine, provides us with the future picture required by faith to materialize.

Here is how it works:

Sometimes young persons in high school have difficulty deciding what course or major subject to pursue in college either because they do not have enough role models to emulate, or do not know enough of the careers and disciplines out there. To help them with these decisions, the school sometimes takes them on excursions or places them on a work study program to help provide them with a picture or model of their possible goals.

In the same way Jesus Christ, the Divine, by his resurrection, provides a glimpse of the universality stage for us to have a picture of our goal and destination after our transition from our physically bound state of existence.

It is interesting to rate that note that Christ was born, lived, and skipped the spiritual stage because He is the Master of that phase. (The reason for phase 2, "Life Begins at Forty," is to become Christ-like.) He went through the Exit Birth phase, which we call death, to show us, in concrete terms, what we would look like after our own "exit birth" into the glory of the universality phase.

One of the major lessons we learned from the life, death, and resurrection of Jesus Christ is that death is not the reason we were born, nor is it the end of our mission.

Because Christ had the picture of His Glorified Self after the resurrection, meaning that He had faith that he would rise from death, he kept his eyes on the ball, so to speak, though like us, He was not particularly thrilled about dying, especially by way of the disgraceful death on the cross.

He sweated blood in distress over his death.

However, he knew that death was neither the end nor the purpose of life, but rather a transition to the universal stage of life and consciousness.

It was his mission to pass through that gate and show us what lies beyond the gate we call death.

His mission was to rise from death and show us the picture of spiritual joy, and the glorified body that is immortal that could come in and out of locked rooms, and could be anywhere, anytime.

After all, that is what we humans all want. Why else do we search for the fountain of youth and resent aging?

Before Christ, we never saw an incorruptible body. Christ's mission was to show us the vision of our ultimate incorruptibility.

LIV

Are you Sure Death is Really Not the End?

Since there would always be skeptics and scientists: there was Thomas, the unbelieving.

Thomas was the epitome of unbelief or lack of faith. He had to see for himself, touch for himself, feel for himself, hear for himself.

Hearsay was not acceptable for Thomas. He wanted hard evidence. Proof.

> Now, Thomas (called Didymus), one of the Twelve, was not with the disciples when Jesus (The Resurrected) came. So the other disciples told him, "We have seen the Lord!"
>
> But he said to them, "Unless I see the nail marks in his hands and put my finger where the nails were, and put my hand into his side, I will not believe it."

A week later his disciples were in the house again, and Thomas was with them. Though the doors wore locked, Jesus came and stood among them and said. "Peace be unto you!" Then he said to Thomas, Put your finger here; see my hands. Reach out your hand and put it into my side. Stop doubting and believe.

Thomas said to him, "My Lord and my God."

Then Jesus told him, "Because you have seen me, you have believed. Blessed are those who have not seen and yet have believed." (John 20:24-29)

No test for physical proof and concretization could be more rigorous than that to which Thomas subjected The Resurrected Christ.

But Jesus did more. He cooked and ate fish and bread with them, not to show that the glorified body would need physical food, but to demonstrate that the glorified body could do anything it wished to do.

Jesus Christ stayed around for forty days after his resurrection to make sure his followers and others got the picture before continuing on His Universality Journey.

Resurrection Picture not Enough for Some People

Despite this picture of the joy of the resurrected Christ, some people still do not believe in life after the so-called death, (which as we now know, is actually the exiting for us into the universality state of life and consciousness.)

This lack of faith by some of these people sometimes make them afraid of the pain of dying. The result is that if they happen to be sick with some painful and disabling disorders, they sometimes opt for direct suicide or assisted suicide.

Ironically, their choice is also an act of faith because they believe that dying will be the end of their consciousness.

Once again like King Solomon, the stock broker and the weather forecaster, they do not know for sure that dying would be the absolute end of their life or sentinel consciousness.

From the tales of near dead experiences that have been gathered so far from people at various stages in their exit route before they reverted to the mortal life, we understand that the majority of people claim that they experience light and a feeling of overwhelming joy as they begin their transition.

However, about eighteen percent of them, according to an A&E (Arts and Entertainment) television documentary in March 2000, are said to report darkness, deep sadness, miserable claustrophobia and general misery and discomfort.

There seems to be much more to these accounts than we currently know.

The beginning of any journey or experience can never quite capture the full journey or experience. Our Earth life experience as infants, for example, cannot be as comprehensive as the story we tell at our ripe wisdom age of eighty or more.

We can therefore only imagine that the accounts given by people with near death experience and even the vivid images of the risen Christ are but a tip of the iceberg of what the real universality journey is like.

Application of our wisdom to these accounts encourage us to keep focused and in tune, and to enjoy the communication channels opened by the spiritual phase two of our life's experience with The Universal Spirit of Creation, God, in preparation for our exit birthing or transition into the third and universal phase of our becoming.

If we do this, we should be happy like larks as we age into our wisdom years.

And if we do not, we should be prepared for the depression of emptiness and nothingness in these precious years. That is not an option for me. How about you?

LV

America Has the Big Picture

You may recall what we said earlier in this book about having a vision for your wisdom years.

We said that what you believe in becomes your future. And what you focus on is what you achieve.

This statement is as true for individual as it is for nations.

History and time have shown that the formulators of the United States of America's Constitution were Men of Wisdom. In birthing the nation, they had the big picture of a successful nation in their minds. They had not traveled that road before, but they had faith. They were not in the future, but they believed in the greatness it held for America

Time has proved them right

At the beginning of the New and Third Millennium of the Resurrected Christ, America was not only a successful world power, it was a formidable economic power.

America was riding the waves of success while other nations crumbled or struggled just to feed themselves and maintain some self respect and dignity. America could do that because it was living the materialization of the faith of the founding fathers.

These sages who formulated the Constitution of the United States of America also nurtured the new nation through its infancy. They knew the value of placing a picture of perfection for the youth to strive toward. They had the wisdom to know that America would probably never attain perfection but that in striving toward it, the nation would overreach every other nation.

When you over reach everyone else, you become number one, imperfect as you may be.

America is today the World's biggest military and economic power because it has kept its faith in and focus on the Maker of power and wealth, God.

Faith requires un-equivocation. America is unequivocal in putting her money where her faith is. "In God we trust." The dollar proclaims this.

In God We Trust

"One Nation Under God."

The dollar proclaims this.

Life is a journey of faith for individuals, nations, corporate bodies and all human institutions. To make it successful, happy and joyous we need the right picture.

> "One nation under God," toward whom, we are all becoming.
>
> Anything else, just won't make it.

References

1. Anderson C, How to Protect Yourself From Memory Loss. *Journal of Longevity,* 2000; Vol. 6, 4: 34-36

2. Avis NE, Sexual Function and Aging in Men and Women: Community and Population based Studies. *Journal of Gender Specific Medicine,* March/ April 2000 Vol. 3, 2: 37-41

3. Baer JW, The Pledge of Allegiance: *A Short History, A Centennial History 1982- 1992,* Annapolis MO. Free State Press, Inc.; 1992

4. Braverman ER, The Pause Model and It's Impact on Health and Disease. PATH Medical Group of New York. 185 Madison Avenue, New York, NY 10016. April 2000.

5. Carlson JE, Role of Physical Activity in the Prevention of Disability for Older Persons. (Institute on Aging, University of Pennsylvania Health System). *Clinical Geriatrics,* March 2000; Vol. 8, 3: 110-1 17

6. Catoir J, The Christophers, Age: Living in the Present Tense. The Christophers News Notes No. 332, February, 1991. 12 East 48th Street, New York, NY 10017

7. Chizea DO, "Link-Up" A New Paradigm for Stress and Stress Management in a New Millennium. *The Mountaineer-Herald,* Ebensburg. PA 1998

8. Chizea DO, Understanding Spirituality: It's Like the Computer. Dora Chizea Productions. Ebensburg. PA 15931. 1999.

9. Chizea DO, Meeting and Knowing Yourself: A One Month Day by Day Program for Self Discovery. Dora Chizea Productions. Ebensburg. PA 15931. 1999

10. Cohen R, Low Testosterone: The Unsuspected Epidemic. Anti-Aging Bulletin, International Antiaging Systems. April - June 2000. Vol. 4, 6: 8- 20.

11. Leni JR, McRae TD, Aricept (donepezil HO) Medicine to Remember, 60. A Collaboration Dedicated to Advances in Alzheimer's Therapy 2000, Esai Inc.* Pfizer Inc., April 2000.

12. Khalsa DS, Cameron S, *Brain Longevity.* Warner Books Inc., 1997,1272 Ave. of Americas, New York, NY 10020.

13. Klatz R, Goldman R, *Stopping The Clock.* Keath Publishing Inc., 27 Pine Street, New Canaan, Connecticut 1996.

14. Stem L, 50 Ways to Save More for Retirement Reader's Digest New Choices (Living Even Better after 5O). Communications Data Services, PO Box 5234, Marian IA 51593 April 2000.

Appendix

Age: Living in the Present Tense

> "This is the day which the Lord has made; Let us rejoice and be glad in it." Psalm 118:24.

When someone told 89-year-old poet Dorothy Duncan that she had lived a full life, she responded tartly, "Don't you past tense me!"

In our youth-oriented society the message often sent to older adults is that their usefulness ends at 65, if not sooner. Many like Dorothy Duncan recognize this for the nonsense it is and go right on leading the productive lives.

* Artist Pablo Picasso was still producing drawing at 90 and his paintings became more innovative with the years.
* Pianist Arthur Rubenstein gave one of his greatest recitals at age 89.
* Actress Jessica Tandy won an Academy Award at 80 for her performance in "Driving Miss Daisy."
* Congressman Claude Pepper of Florida was still actively championing the rights of the elderly and the poor at the age of 88.
* Environmental Marjory Stoneman Douglas, credited with saving the Everglades, is still fighting for the cause at age 100.

Happy, productive older people don't necessarily refuse to retire from their jobs. But they do refuse to retire from life.

Enjoying the Freedom

According to a 1989 *Los Angeles Times* poll, nearly two-thirds of Americans 65 and over are happy with their lives. Only half of those 18 to 49 are happy. Age clearly has something going for it. One advantage is increased freedom:

* Freedom to enjoy special interests: Isidore Moskowhz had no time for hobbies during the years he and his wife worked long hours in their Brooklyn ice cream parlor and brought up their children. He first tried painting at the age of 70. At 86 he had a one-man show in Madison Avenue gallery.
* Freedom to set your own goals and pace: After raising four sons, Lena Genser of Jersey City had a chance to continue her own education. Working at her own pace, she finished high school, obtained a college degree at age 83, and took up computer programming at 90.
* Freedom to reach out: Constance Daniels, 91, collects and distributes tons of clothing and household hems to Milwaukee's poor. This clothing has helped so many people feel more comfortable at school or job interviews that she has been called "a worker of minor miracles."

Recognizing Opportunities

In addition to more freedom, the later years can bring exciting opportunities:

* Second careers: Artist and retired teacher Nola Denslo is busy with another career at 87. She runs a non profit arts education center for the frail elderly in Lamoille County, Vermont. Students, who range in age from 69 to 97, are winning prizes, selling art, and getting books published.

* When New York fireman John Burke retired, he studied nursing and now assists at operations. Burke's work as a firefighter involved first aid, and nursing appealed to him as a way to continue helping save lives.
* Volunteer work: George Sable, a retired engineer in his late 70s, designs equipment for the disabled. His volunteer work began when he designed a hand-pedaled bike for disabled children in Minneapolis. "The smiles on these kids' faces," he said, "that's all I needed."
* Hobbies: Former New York social worker Fannie White found a way to combine a hobby with volunteer work. At age 94 she started a stamp club for fifth graders, using stamps to tutor them in history and geography.
* Sports: The Over the Hill Gang ski club requires that members be at least 50. Don't be fooled by the name. The group's motto is, "Once you're over the hill, you pick up speed." Another group, the 70+ Ski club, has members in their 70s, 80s and 90s.
* Retired real estate investor Eric de Reynier, of Albany, California, took up hang gliding when he was 72. He was still at it in his 80s. Hulda Crooks, of Loma Linda, California, climbed Mount Whitney for the 23rd time at age 90.
* Education: Robert Fleming of Little Rock studied computer science, piano, and politics in an Elderhostel program. Elderhostel offers people 60 or older one-week courses at colleges in the U.S. and abroad. "It gets the cobwebs out of your mind," said Fleming.

Dealing with Problems

Older adults do have to deal with some special problems. Among them are negative stereotypes concerns about health, loneliness and finances.

....negative stereotypes

We're led to believe that old people are feeble, forgetful, and senile. So as we get older, we begin looking for signs that we're falling apart At age 20 misplacing a pair of glasses isn't evidence of mental deterioration. At age 80 it still isn't.

People are conditioned to believe that 65 equals uselessness, said Dr. Gustave Eckstein, who began learning Russian at 85 when he was writing a book about Pavlov. If we're told something often enough, he said, we believe it whether it makes sense or not.

These stereotypes are being challenged.

Twenty years ago, after Maggie Kuhn was forced to retire at 65, she founded the Gray Panthers to champion the rights of older people. She's still active in its work. She says she would like her epitaph to read, "Here lies Maggie, under the only stone she ever left unturned."

Growing in numbers and purchasing power, older citizens are making their influence felt. Advertisers are beginning to show older people in a more positive light. One commercial features 72-year-old Lena Horne. The glamorous singer clearly doesn't belong in a rocking chair.

...health

Many problems once thought to be caused by age are really caused by poor health habits. A balanced diet and regular exercise can improve health at any age. One group of 70-year-old men who took part in an exercise program had the bodily reactions of men of 40 at the end of the year.

At 82 Eula Weaver suffered from angina, congestive heart failure, high blood pressure, and arthritis. At 85, after three years of careful diet and exercise, she won two gold medals in the Senior Olympics.

Even with serious health problems, life can be productive and happy.

When French Artist Auguste Renoir was 60, his fingers were too stiff for him to hold a brush and he was unable to walk. He worked with a brush strapped to his wrist and continued to paint for 18 years.

At age 100, Iva Blake had one of the most beautiful gardens in Albuquerque. She gardened from a wheel chair, using special tools.

Faith in God and a sense of humor help. At age 80 President John Quincy Adams, when asked how he was, replied,

> "Mr Adams is quite alright, thank you. Of course, the house he lives in is a bit dilapidated; its walls are tottering on their foundations; its roof is greatly in need of repair. I think he is soon going to have to move out of his old house into another not made with hands. However, Mr. Adams is quite all right, thank you."

...loneliness

Retirement can mean losing touch with long-time fellow workers. And as the years bring the death of old friends, making new ones can be hard, especially in cities.

Senior citizens' centers offer a good way to meet people. So do churches and synagogues. Some even have special activities for older members. Helping others also helps ward off loneliness.

In the New York restaurant they run, Jeanette Le Pourhiet and Madeleine Ribes, both over 65, often have fund raisers to help AIDS victims and others in need. The widowed Mrs. Le Pourhiet says, "I'm not really alone because this is my life."

At age 78 Winifred Nazarian of New Jersey does volunteer work at a nursing home one day a week. She says, "If you stay home alone, self pity, the big enemy, will creep in."

...finances

Some retirees feel the pinch of living on a reduced income. The cost of housing in particular may be a problem.

Walter Smith, 77 year old widower, found upkeep and taxes on his large Vermont farmhouse alarming, and he didn't like living alone. Project SHARE, a Vermont program that matches elderly people who have extra space with those who need a place to live, arranged for four people to share his house. He now has money for repairs and enjoys having people around.

Senior citizen discounts and special considerations from government agencies and utilities can help financially. And free movies, concerts, and lectures offered by public libraries are a real boon.

Lots of people supplement retirement income by part-time work. Employers often prefer older workers for part-time jobs, finding their maturity and dependability to be valuable assets.

Retired children's librarian Ellie Gibbs, 78, now works part-time at a school library. She finds the extra money helpful and loves the work. She says she's being "recycled."

Growing in Love and Faith

When poet Mary Sarton was in her 60s, she wrote:

> "If the whole of life is a journey toward old age, then I believe it is also a journey toward love...Old age is not

an illness; it is a timeless ascent. As power diminishes we grow toward more light."

There is a growing concern for others in the middle age and after, psychologists tell us. This reaching out takes many forms.

Zenaida Corpuz of Chicago worked as a nurse while she brought up her children. When the youngest graduated from college, Ms. Corpuz, 55, volunteered for work at a mission clinic in Chile. She says, "Now it is my turn to give something back for the many blessings I received."

There is also growing closeness to God. Later life can be a time of spiritual growth, of seeing things in a clearer perspective.

Eugene Bianchi, author of *Aging as a Spiritual Journey,* said, "It is only when you begin to count your years from the end rather than the beginning that you begin to ask the deeper questions about what should be done with the time remaining."

In his book, *Say Yes to Life,* Rabbi Sidney Greenberg calls time the thoughtful thief, because for everything it steals from us, it gives us something in return.

"While time was stealing the smoothness from our skins," says Rabbi Greenberg, "it was giving us the opportunity to remove the wrinkles from our souls."

"There is a difference between getting older and growing into old age," wrote Presbyterian minister Carl Wolf, in *Fellowship in Prayer* magazine. "Some individuals in their mature years bog down in nostalgia, remembering...the past...others...enter the way of spiritual pilgrimage...For these, the maturing years offer a wonderful adventure with the spirit of God."

This pilgrimage helps me to answer the questions, "Who am I?" and "Who am I becoming?"

Spiritual sharing grows apace.

> After retirement, former Memphis attorney Frank Miles spent much of his time in lay ministry to the sick. He found that the work begins "a deep satisfaction at having used your time to help someone in need."
>
> Mary Baker Eddy, founder of the Christian Science Church, was still directing it at 89.
>
> Pope John XXIII became the pope at the age of 77. His dynamic leadership set in motion Vatican Council II, which brought important changes to the Catholic Church, and he became a light to the world.
>
> In his book *Life in the Afternoon,* Edward Fischer says, "To be alive means that you still have a part to play in the magnificent drama. You are still needed."

SO TEACH US TO NUMBER OUR DAYS THAT WE MAY GET A HEART OF WISDOM. (PS. 90:12)

Grow old along with me!

The best is yet to be,

The last of life,

for which the first was made.

Our times are in his hand

Who saith, "A whole I planned;

Youth shows but half.

Trust God: see all, nor be afraid!"

—Robert Browning.

Aging: The Myths...the Realities

Myths: Mental ability declines with age.

Reality: People who continue to use their minds, to have absorbing interests, don't decline in intellectual ability unless they suffer from a condition such as a Alzheimer's disease.

Myth: Memory grows poorer as we grow older.

Reality: In their 70s most people experience some drop in ability to remember recent events. But other types of memory; for knowledge and facts and skills; are not affected by age.

Myth: Age brings serious health problems.

Reality: Many people enjoy good health in later life. Hearing and vision dim and the reflexes slow. But lots of other problems attributed to aging are not related to age. Proper diet and exercise can help prevent or reverse conditions such as high blood pressure and osteoporosis.

Myth: Retirement age was set at 65 because job performance is poor after 65. Reality: There was no relationship when German Chancellor Otto von Bismarck set up the first socialistic labor standards by giving workers benefits. He chose 65 as the age to begin pension payments because few Germans then lived much past 65! Other nations later used the age set by Germany.

Resources and Referrals

Vitamin Research Products 3579 Highway 50 East Carson City, NV 89701 Tel: 800-877-2447 www.VRP.com
Robert Watson, President
Tel: 775-887-7518

FABOG Services
Vitamin and Natural Products Distributors
1622 Miriam Court
Elmont, NY 11003
Tel: 516-825-0555
wwwJABOO@AOL.COM

Stress Management & Anti-Aging Group
262 Lincoln Street, Ebensburg, PA 15931
Tel/ Fax: 814-472-4294
E-mail: Dora@Cambrianews.com
Source of Speakers for Lectures, Seminars and Workshops on The Stresses of Life and Anti-Aging Medicine

Index

T

U

V

W